Current Topics in Microbiology 140 and Immunology

Editors

R.W. Compans, Birmingham/Alabama · M. Cooper,
Birmingham/Alabama · H. Koprowski, Philadelphia
I. McConell, Edinburgh · F. Melchers, Basle
M. Oldstone, La Jolla/California · S. Olsnes, Oslo
H. Saedler, Cologne · P.K. Vogt, Los Angeles
H. Wagner, Munich · I. Wilson, La Jolla/California

Cytotoxic Effector Mechanisms

Edited by E.R. Podack

With 24 Figures

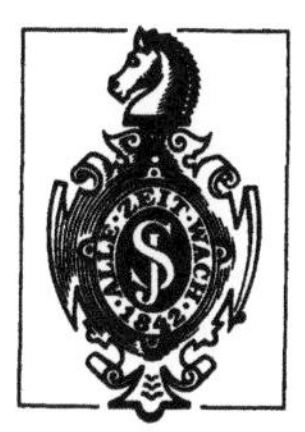

Springer-Verlag
Berlin Heidelberg New York
London Paris Tokyo

Eckhard R. Podack, M.D.
Department of Microbiology and Immunology
University of Miami School of Medicine
P.O. Box 016960 (R-138)
Miami, FL 33101
USA

ISBN-13: 978-3-642-73913-2   e-ISBN-13: 978-3-642-73911-8
DOI: 10.1007/978-3-642-73911-8

© Springer-Verlag Berlin Heidelberg 1989
Library of Congress Catalog Card Number 15-12910
Softcover reprint of the hardcover 1st edition 1989

2123/3130-543210 – Printed on acid-free paper

Table of Contents

E.R. PODACK: Granule-Mediated Cytolysis
of Target Cells
With 1 Figure   1

E.R. PODACK, K.J. OLSEN, D.M. LOWREY,
and M.G. LICHTENHELD:
Structure and Function of Perforin   11

J.M. SODETZ: Structure and Function of C8 in the
Membrane Attack Sequence of Complement
With 2 Figures   19

D.E. JENNE and J. TSCHOPP: Granzymes: a Family
of Serine Proteases in Granules of Cytolytic T
Lymphocytes
With 3 Figures   33

K.K. STANLEY: The Molecular Mechanism
of Complement C9 Insertion and Polymerisation
in Biological Membranes
With 5 Figures   49

R.C. BLEACKLEY: The Isolation and Characterization
of Two Cytotoxic T-Lymphocyte-Specific Serine
Protease Genes
With 1 Figure   67

R.J. HERSHBERGER, C. MUELLER, H.K. GERSHENFELD,
and I.L. WEISSMAN: A Serine Protease-Encoding
Gene That Marks Activated Cytotoxic T Cells
In Vivo and In Vitro
With 2 Figures   81

R.L. STEVENS, M.N. KAMADA, and W.E. SERAFIN:
Structure and Function of the Family of Proteoglycans That Reside in the Secretory Granules
of Natural Killer Cells and Other Effector Cells
of the Immune Response
With 4 Figures   93

VI   Table of Contents

G. HAENSCH: The Homologous Species Restriction
   of the Complement Attack: Structure and Function
   of the C8 Binding Protein
   With 6 Figures 109

Subject Index 119

Indexed in Current Contents

List of Contributors

You will find the addresses at the beginning of the respective contribution

BLEACKLEY, R.C.   67

GERSHENFELD, H.K.   81

HAENSCH, G. 109

HERSHBERGER, R.J.   81

JENNE, D.E.   33

KAMADA, M.N.   93

LICHTENHELD, M.G.   11

LOWREY, D.M.   11

MUELLER, C.   81

OLSEN, K.J.   11

PODACK, E.R.   1, 11

SERAFIN, W.E.   93

SODETZ, J.M.   19

STANLEY, K.K.   49

STEVENS, R.L.   93

TSCHOPP, J.   33

WEISSMAN, I.L.   81

Granule-Mediated Cytolysis of Target Cells

E.R. PODACK

1   Introduction 1
2   The Hypothesis of Vectorial Granule Secretion in Cell Lysis 1
3   Properties of Isolated Cytolytic Granules from T and NK Cells 2
4   The Role of Perforin 1 in Granule-Mediated Lysis 3
4.1 Perforins Are Not the Sole Effectors of Cell-Mediated Lysis 4
5   Factors Causing DNA Degradation: Delivery Through P1? 4
5.1 P1-Mediated Delivery of Factors 5
5.2 Effect of Intracellular Ca Chelation 5
5.3 Other Granule Factors 6
6   Controversies 7
7   Perspective 7
References 7

1 Introduction

The lysis of target cells attacked by cytotoxic T cells appears to be caused by two possibly related phenomena, namely the formation of transmembrane pores in the target cell's membrane and the cleavage and release of the target cell's nuclear DNA. At present it is not entirely clear how these effects are mediated at a molecular level. However, in the past few years, concepts have evolved and been experimentally tested that allow the formulation of a comprehensive hypothesis to explain the main steps of lymphocyte-mediated cytolysis (PODACK 1985; HENKART 1985). This said, it should be pointed out, however, that at the time of writing none of the effector molecules discussed below can be unequivocally linked to the cytolytic process, when intact killer cells lyse a target cell.

2 The Hypothesis of Vectorial Granule Secretion in Cell Lysis

Killer cells recognize their targets through specific membrane adhesion proteins. Recognition is followed by the formation of conjugates between killer and target

Department of Microbiology and Immunology, University of Miami School of Medicine, Miami, FL 33101, USA

Current Topics in Microbiology and Immunology, Vol. 140
© Springer-Verlag Berlin · Heidelberg 1988

cell. It is likely that the engagement of cell surface receptors of the killer cell transmits transmembrane signals leading to the activation of its secretory machinery. This process is accompanied by a wave of Ca fluxes traversing the killer cell from its distal end (opposite the conjugation site) to the proximal end. Simultaneously, the killer cell undergoes a reorientation in such a way that its Golgi apparatus, the microtubule organization center (MTOC), and cytoplasmic granules become oriented towards the conjugation site (KUPFER et al. 1985; GEIGER et al. 1982; YANNELLI et al. 1986). Killer cell reorientation is absolutely required for target cell lysis. Reorientation may proceed even in the absence of extracellular Ca (OSTERGAARD and CLARK 1987). However, it is blocked by tubulin blockers, resulting in inhibition of lysis. Subsequent to reorientation, individual granules of the killer cell are vectorially secreted in the direction of the target conjugation site (PODACK and DENNERT 1983). This entire process requires between 5 and 15 min at 37° C. Following granule secretion, the actual cell death of the target cell, as measured by ^{51}Cr or DNA release proceeds within the next one-half to several hours.

These briefly sketched events are supported by numerous morphological studies, by studies using metabolic blockers of secretion and of cytoskeletal elements (KUPFER et al. 1985), by Ca flux measurements with fluorescent dyes (IMBODEN and STOBO 1985), and by the measurement of the release during cytolysis of granule markers (SCHMIDT et al. 1985; TAKAYAMA et al. 1987).

3 Properties of Isolated Cytolytic Granules from T and NK Cells (Table 1)

Perhaps the strongest supportive evidence for the secretory model of lymphocyte-mediated cytolysis comes from the functional analysis of isolated cytolytic granules (HENKART et al. 1984; PODACK and KONIGSBERG 1984):

Table 1. Functional properties of cytolytic granules

Source: murine T-cells
Kinetics of lysis: rapid (2 min, 37° C)
Ion requirements: Ca(Sr)
Target specificity: none (all targets are lysed)
Inhibitors of rapid lysis: (a) Zn ions, (b) serum (lipoproteins, S-protein), (c) preincubation with Ca
Activity after preincubation with Ca: slow L-cell lysis (24–28 h)

Granules are obtained from cloned killer cells by nitrogen cavitation and subsequent Percoll gradient fractionation of the postnuclear cell lysate in the presence of ethylene glycol tetra-acetic acid (EGTA). Under these conditions, granules sediment to the dense region of the gradient, representing a virtually homogeneous subcellular fraction. Granules isolated in this way are highly cytotoxic for all target cells. Granule-mediated cytolysis is dependent on Ca ions and elevated temperature (37° C). Lysis is exceedingly rapid and essentially complete within 2 min at 37° C. If serum is added during the lytic stage, granule-mediated lysis is strongly inhibited. The inhibition of serum is largely due to serum lipoproteins and to S-protein. Preincubation of granules for 5 min in the presence of Ca or Zn at 37° C also abrogates their cytolytic activity. Intracellularly, Ca is excluded from granules even during cell activation and increase of intracellular Ca.

It is thus clear that granules, if involved as effectors for cell-mediated cytolysis, must be protected from serum as well as from premature exposure to Ca ions. These conditions are presumably met at the killer target conjugation site. In all likelihood, granules are secreted into the interstitial space of the contact zone which probably excludes plasma proteins and may also regulate the flux of Ca ions.

4 The Role of Perforin 1 in Granule-Mediated Lysis (Table 2)

Virtually all the *rapid* lytic effects of granules described above can be explained by the presence in the granules of one protein, perforin 1 (P1) (DENNERT and PODACK 1983; PODACK and DENNERT 1983), also known as cytolysin:

Table 2. Functional properties of perforin (P1)

Source: murine T-cell granules
Kinetics of lysis: rapid (2 min, 37° C),
Ion requirements: Ca
Target specificity: none
Inhibitors: (a) Zn ions, (b) serum, (c) preincubation with Ca
Activity after preincubation with Ca: none

P1 is a Ca-dependent, pore-forming protein of 70 K–75 K (PODACK et al. 1985; MASSON and TSCHOPP 1985). Similar to complement component C9, pore formation of P1 results from the polymerization of approximately 20 molecules into a hollow tubular complex with amphiphilic properties. The polymerization reaction is both temperature and Ca dependent, a corollary to the properties of granule-mediated lysis. The amphiphilic character of poly P1 is also a consequence of P1-polymerization. During polymerization, globular P1 unfolds into an elongated molecule, exposing a previously hidden hydrophobic domain. If this process occurs on a target membrane, P1 inserts into the membrane, where the Ca-dependent polymerization proceeds and a transmembrane channel is formed.

Polymerized P1 in membranes is detectable under the electron microscope as a 16 nm wide transmembrane tubule. A whole spectrum of functional channel sizes ranging from 1–16 nm are measured as conductance increase across planar lipid bilayers upon addition of purified P1 to the conductance chamber (YOUNG et al. 1986). The smaller channel sizes are thought to be caused by P1 oligomers ranging from $P1_2$ to $P1_{\sim 20}$. It is important to remember that the effects of P1 can be mediated in the absence of electron microscopically detectable circular lesions which are only formed by $P1_{\sim 20}$.

As mentioned above for granules, P1 is also inhibited by serum and by preincubation with Ca. Inhibition is caused by different mechanisms: Serum lipoproteins provide membrane analogues for P1 insertion and thus may compete with target membranes. Ca, on the other hand, allows P1 polymerization in the fluid phase. Polymerized P1 is not capable of inserting into membranes: Unfolding through polymerization and membrane insertion have to be coordinated processes.

4.1   Perforins Are Not the Sole Effectors of Cell-Mediated Lysis

The foregoing description indicates that all the rapid effects observed in granule-mediated lysis appear to be caused by their content of P1. In particular, the rapid lysis by granules of tumor cells and of erythrocytes, accompanied by the formation of transmembrane pores, certainly is caused by P1. However, the DNA degradation in target cells, which is observed when intact killer cells lyse them, is not readily explainable with P1. In fact, evidence has already been presented in early studies by Russel (RUSSEL and DOBOS 1980) that pore formation by complement does not cause DNA degradation (however, see also SHIPLEY et al. 1971). Similarly, pore formation by isolated P1 may not trigger DNA degradation. Preincubation of granules with Ca ions eliminates P1 activity due to P1 polymerization. Nevertheless, P1-inactivated granules still lyse L cells (both TNF-sensitive and TNF-resistant lines). This L-cell lysis is a slow process requiring 24–48 h (Table 3). The slow lytic activity appears to be responsible

Table 3. Properties of nucleolysis triggering factors

Parameter	Murine NTF	Human NTF
Source	CTL	IL2-activated cells (14 days) (LANK)
Molecular weight	68 K	?
Target	L929	K 562, Daudi, Raji
Time course	> 18 h	> 3 h
P1 dependence	No	No
Ca dependence	ND	Yes
DNA degradation	+ (?)	ND
Inhibition by:		
anti-TNF	10%–40%	ND
anti-LT	No	ND
anti-granules	Yes	ND

NTF, nucleolysis triggering factors; *ND*, no data

for DNA degradation in the target cell (KONIGSBERG and PODACK 1985; KONIGSBERG and PODACK 1986; LIU et al. 1987).

5   Factors Causing DNA Degradation: Delivery Through P1?

The role of DNA degradation in cell death has been studied in various systems including hormone-induced cell death (RUSSEL and DOBOS 1980; DUKE et al. 1983; UCKER 1987; SCHMID et al. 1986; DUKE et al. 1986). The main difference between hormone- and T-cell-induced DNA degradation is the fact that the former requires target cell protein synthesis whereas the latter does not. The ultimate DNA cleavage is executed by a target enzyme. How does the killer lymphocyte trigger DNA degradation? Two competing models have been proposed:

1. The push-button hypothesis of DNA degradation. According to this model, the killer cell triggers, by binding to the target, a suicidal pathway in the target cell. No specific factor is delivered by the killer or taken up by the target in this model.

2. The uptake hypothesis of DNA degradation. In this model, the killer cell manufactures and delivers a factor that is taken up by the target cell and triggers an intracellular target cell pathway resulting in DNA degradation. Uptake of this putative factor could be mediated through specific target cell receptor-mediated entry or through nonspecific (P1) mediated delivery via transmembrane pores and endocytosis.

5.1 P1-Mediated Delivery of Factors

Transmembrane pores are strong signals for endocytosis. In particular, studies by CARNEY et al. (1985) have demonstrated that transmembrane pores are removed from the cell membrane by endocytosis, a pathway considered as membrane repair. Stimulation of endocytosis by pores in turn is dependent on the Ca flux through these pores into the target cell. In the absence of extracellular Ca, and hence in the absence of transmembrane Ca fluxes, neither membrane repair nor pore removal through endocytosis takes place.

From these known facts it is safe to assume that whenever P1 is delivered and in a Ca-dependent process polymerized into pores on a target membrane, active endocytotic repair processes will ensue. This endocytotic process by necessity will engulf into endosomes material previously secreted together with P1 (pinocytosis). Thus, if granules contain factors responsible for nucleolytic breakdown of DNA (nucleolysis triggering factors, NTF), they could conveniently enter the target cell through the P1-mediated delivery, i.e., by P1-triggered endocytosis.

5.2 Effect of Intracellular Ca Chelation

If target cells are loaded with an intracellular Ca chelator, DNA degradation is completely abrogated, whereas ^{51}Cr release is slightly increased (Fig. 1). This finding allows several possible explanations, three of which are discussed:

1. The suicidal pathway resulting in DNA degradation requires available intracellular Ca.
2. NTF-receptor (if existent)-mediated uptake is blocked by intracellular Ca chelation.
3. NTF delivery through P1-mediated endocytosis is blocked by intracellular Ca chelation.

The fact that ^{51}Cr release increases in targets pretreated with intracellular Ca chelators is consistent with the lack of removal of P1 channels. This may

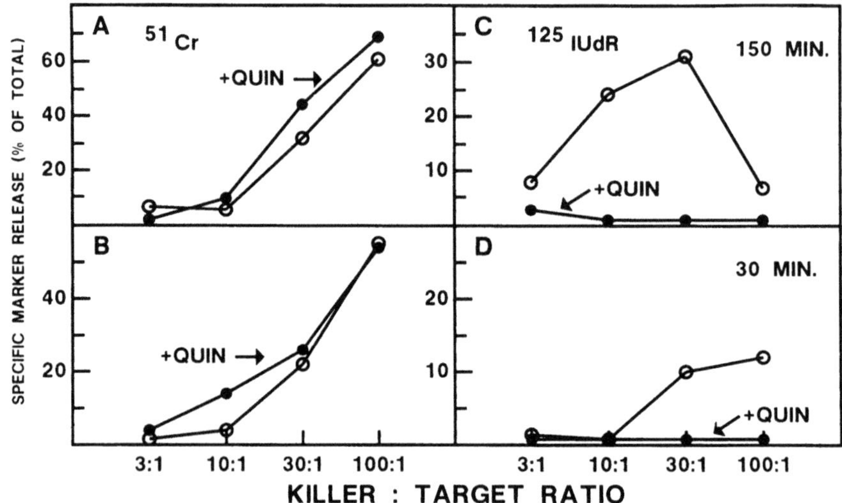

Fig. 1A–D. Inhibition of DNA release and enhancement of Cr release by loading of target cells with Quin2, an intracellular Ca chelator (0.8 mM intracellular concentration). The target cells were EL4 and the killer cells human LAK cells after 2 weeks activation with 500 U/ml r-IL2. ●–● targets with Quin2; o–o targets without Quin2. **A, B** ^{51}Cr release at 150 min (**A**) and 30 min (**B**). **C, D** ^{125}IUdR release at 150 min (**C**) and 30 min (**D**)

be taken as evidence for the absence of repair through endocytosis similar to experiments of complement repair. The block of endocytosis may result in the failure of pinocytotic NTF uptake into endosomes and in the failure to trigger DNA degradation.

One other important conclusion can be drawn from the experiment in Fig. 1. Even though DNA degradation is completely blocked, cell lysis proceeds. DNA degradation thus is not essential for cell death as mediated by killer lymphocytes (HOWELL and MARTZ 1987). Does DNA degradation promote and enhance cell death? This is entirely possible. The fact that Ca deletion stabilizes P1 channels and enhances P1-mediated lysis could obscure the contribution of DNA degradation to cell lysis.

Particularly at low doses of P1 (3:1 killer:target), which may not be sufficient to kill a target cell, the uptake of NTF and DNA degradation could be important. In fact, under these conditions, the observed DNA degradation is maximal. At high doses of P1, such as will be delivered at 100:1 killer:target ratio, P1 alone appears to be responsible for cell death, and DNA degradation is minimal (Fig. 1; DUKE et al. 1986). These findings are entirely consistent with the NTF uptake model mediated nonspecifically by P1-triggered endocytosis.

5.3 Other Granule Factors

Granules contain chondroitin sulfate whose function may be to package granule factors. In addition, chondroitin sulfate may furnish the killer cell membrane at the contact site with a protective layer. Chondroitin sulfate, similar to heparin, inhibits P1 activity and thus may protect the killer cell from its own cytolytic molecules (see p. 93–108; STEVENS et al., this volume).

By far the largest portion of granule proteins is accounted for by proteolytic enzymes. The function and structure of these enzymes are discussed in detail in other chapters of this book (see p. 33–47; JENNE and TSCHOPP).

6 Controversies

Peritoneal exudate cells (PEL) are primarily MHC-restricted cytotoxic T cells. These cells have very low (DENNERT and PODACK 1983; MUNGER et al. 1987) or undetectable levels of granules and P1 (DENNERT et al. 1987; BERKE and ROSEN 1987). It has, therefore, been suggested (BERKE and ROSEN 1987) that in vivo-generated (CTL may have a killing mechanism different from in vitro-cultured cells. We have found (E.R. PODACK, H. HENGARTNER, unpublished data) that in vivo-generated LCMV-specific CTL contain P1 mRNA, and thus there does not seem to be a difference between virus-specific CTL generated in vivo or in vitro.

Certain target cells are lysed in the absence of extracellular Ca ions and without detectable release of BLT-esterase (a granule marker) (OSTERGAARD et al. 1987; TRENN et al. 1987). These observations have been used to question the validity of the hypothesis of granule-mediated cytolysis.

Before drawing conclusions from these observations, consider the following:
1. It is entirely possible that two independent pathways of target cell lysis may be operative. In fact, the demonstration of lymphotoxin secretion by CTL suggests a granule-independent pathway, because lymphotoxin does not seem to be localized in granules.
2. The presence of a factor causing DNA degradation in target cells that seems to be partly localized in the granules raises the possibility that granules may be endowed with two types of killer molecules which may operate under different circumstances independently of each other.
3. The factors such as P1 and NTF may be organized both in vesicles and in granules. During the induction phase, it is likely that these factors are

Table 4. Properties of granules from various cells[a]

Name	Type	Antigen dependent	Hemolysis	P1 antigen	P1 message	P1 independent cell lysis	Esterase
CTLL2	CTL-NK	No	+ + +	+ + +	ND	+	+ + +
HY3AG	CTL-NK	No	+ + +	+ + +	+ + +	+	+ + +
8–10	CTL	Yes	+	+	+ +	ND	ND
21C11	Helper	Yes	−	+	+ +	ND	+ +
LANK[b]	NK	No	−	+ +	+ +	+ +	+ + +

ND, no data
[a] See note added in proof
[b] IL2-activated human killer cells. Bulk cultures after 2 weeks of IL2 activation, approximately 60% Leu11-positive. All other cells are cloned cells of murine origin

associated with vesicles and have not been organized and stored in the form of granules. PEL, for instance, develop granules only after several days of culture in lymphokine-containing medium, simultaneously appreciably increasing in cytolytic activity.
4. The induction and level of P1 and NTF may vary. We, and others, have observed that granules isolated from different clones and cell lines vary considerably in their hemolytic activity (Table 4); this may be a reflection of differing P1 levels.

7 Perspective

The investigation of the structural and functional properties of cytolytic granules has allowed the formulation of new concepts for the molecular mechanism of lymphocyte-mediated cytolysis. These new concepts led to a renaissance of interest in this challenging field. More importantly, however, this research has given us the biochemical tools to evaluate critically the hypotheses discussed in this and other chapters and to address still controversial areas in the mechanism of cell-mediated cytotoxicity.

Note added in proof:
Since submission of this manuscript we have found that hemolytically active perforin can be obtained from inactive granules by salt extraction in both the human and murine system; see LICHTENHELD et al., Nature, in press (1988)

References

Berke G, Rosen D (1987) Are lytic granules and perforin 1 thereof involved in lysis induced by in vivo primed, peritoneal exudate CTL? Transplant Proc 19:412

Carney DF, Koski CL, Shin ML (1985) Elimination of terminal complement intermediates from the plasma membrane of nucleated cells: the rate of disappearance differs for cells carrying C5b-7 or C5b-8 or a mixture of C5b-8 with a limited number of C5b-9. J Immunol 134:1804

Dennert G, Podack ER (1983) Cytolysis by H2 specific T-killer cells: assembly of tubular complexes during the lytic reaction. J Exp Med 157:1483–1495

Dennert G, Anderson CG, Psocharka G (1987) High activity of Nα-benzyloxycarbonyl-L-lysine thiobenzylester serine esterase and cytolytic perforin in cloned cell lines is not demonstrable in vivo-induced cytotoxic effector cells. Proc Natl Acad Sci USA 84:5004

Duke RL, Chervenak R, Cohen JJ (1983) Endogenous endonuclease-induced DNA fragmentation: an early event in cell-mediated cytolysis. Proc Natl Acad Sci USA 80:6361

Duke RC, Cohen JJ, Chervenak R (1986) Differences in target cell DNA fragmentation induced by mouse cytotoxic T lymphocytes and natural killer cells. J Immunol 137:1442

Geiger B, Rosen D, Berke G (1982) Spatial relationships of MTOC and the contact area of CTLs and target cells. J Cell Biol 95:137

Henkart PA (1985) Mechanism of lymphocyte-mediated cytotoxicity. Annu Rev Immunol 3:31–58

Henkart P, Millard P, Reynolds C, Henkart M (1984) Cytolytic activity of purified cytoplasmic granules from cytotoxic rat LGL tumors. J Exp Med 160:75

Howell DM, Martz E (1987) The degree of CTL-induced DNA solubilization is not determined by the human vs. mouse origin of the target cell. J Immunol 138:2087

Imboden JB, Stobo JD (1985) Transmembrane signalling by the T-cell antigen receptor. Perturbation of T3-antigen receptor complex generates inositol phosphates and releases calcium ions from intracellular stores. J Exp Med 161:446

Konigsberg PJ, Podack ER (1986) DNA damage of target cells by cytolytic T-cell granules. J Cell Biochem [Suppl] 10B:85

Konigsberg PY, Podack ER (1985) Target cell DNA-fragmentation induced by cytolytic T-cell granules. J Leukocyte Biol 38:109

Kupfer A, Dennert G, Singer SJ (1985) The reorientation of the Golgi apparatus and the MTOC in the cytotoxic effector cell is a prerequisite in the lysis of bound target cells. J Mol Cell Immunol 2:37

Liu CC, Steffen M, King F, Young JDE (1987) Identification, isolation, and characterization of a novel cytotoxin in murine cytolytic lymphocytes. Cell 51:393

Masson D, Tschopp J (1985) Isolation of a lytic, pore-forming protein (perforin) from cytolytic T-lymphocytes. J Biol Chem 260:9069

Munger WE, Berrelei G, Henkart PH (1987) Granule exocytosis by cytotoxic T-lymphocytes generated in vivo. Ann Inst Pasteur 138:301

Ostergaard H, Clark WR (1987) The role of Ca in activation of mature cytotoxic T-lymphocytes for lysis. J Immunol 139:3573

Ostergaard HL, Kane KP, Mescher MI, Clark WR (1987) Cytotoxic T lymphocyte-mediated lysis without release of serine esterase. Nature 330:71

Podack ER (1985) The molecular mechanism of lymphocyte-mediated tumor cell lysis. Immunol Today 6:21–27

Podack ER, Dennert G (1983) Cell mediated cytolysis: assembly of two types of tubules with putative cytolytic function by cloned natural killer cells. Nature 302:442–445

Podack ER, Konigsberg PJ (1984) Cytolytic T-cell granules. Isolation, structural, biochemical, and functional characterization. J Exp Med 160:695

Podack ER, Young JDE, Cohn ZA (1985) Isolation and biochemical and functional characterization of perforin 1 from cytolytic T-cell granules. Proc Natl Acad Sci USA 82:8629

Russel JH, Dobos CB (1980) Mechanism of immune lysis. II. CTL-induced nuclear disintegration begins within minutes of cell contact. J Immunol 125:1256

Schmid DS, Tite JP, Ruddle NM (1986) DNA fragmentation: manifestation of target cell destruction mediated by cytotoxic T-cell lines, lymphotoxin-secreting helper T-cell clones, and cell-free lymphotoxin-containing supernatant. Proc Natl Acad Sci USA 83:1881

Schmidt RE, MacDermott RP, Bartley G, Bertovitch M, Amato DA, Austen KF, Schlossman SF, Stevens RL, Ritz J (1985) Specific release of proteoglycans from human natural killer cells during target cell lysis. Nature 318:289

Shipley WU, Baker AR, Colten H (1971) DNA degradation in mammalian cells following complement mediated cytolysis. J Immunol 106:576

Takayama M, Trenn G, Humphrey W, Bluestone J, Henkart P, Sitkovsky M (1987) Antigen receptor triggered secretion of a trypsin like esterase from cytotoxic T-lymphocytes. J Immunol 138:566

Trenn G, Takayama H, Sitkovsky MV (1987) Exocytosis of cytolytic granules may not be required for target cell lysis by cytotoxic T-lymphocytes. Nature 330:72

Ucker D (1987) Cytotoxic T lymphocytes and glucocorticoids activate an endogenous suicide process in target cells. Nature 327:62

Yannelli JR, Sullivan JA, Mandel GL, Engelhard VM (1986) Reorientation and fusion of cytotoxic T-lymphocyte granules after interaction with target cells as determined by high resolution cinemicrography. J Immunol 136:377

Young JDE, Cohn ZA, Podack ER (1986) The ninth component of cytotoxic T-cells: structural and functional homologies. Science 233:184–190

Structure and Function of Perforin

E.R. PODACK, K.J. OLSEN, D.M. LOWREY, and M. LICHTENHELD

1 Introduction and Historical Aspects   11
2 The Poly Perforin Complex   12
3 Isolation and Properties of Perforin   12
4 The Structure of Perforin   13
5 Human Perforin   14
6 Perforin-mRNA Expression   14
References   16

1 Introduction and Historical Aspects

The most striking aspect of lymphocyte-mediated cytolysis is the formation of membrane lesions on target membranes as first described by DOURMASHKIN et al. (1980). In these early studies, a mixed population of effector cells was used, leaving open the question as to whether the observed membrane lesions were in fact assembled by cytotoxic lymphocytes. Subsequent studies by Podack and Dennert using clonal populations of cytotoxic effector lymphocytes demonstrated that the membrane lesions in fact arose from precursor molecules contained in cloned natural Killer (NK) and T cells (DENNERT and PODACK 1983; PODACK and DENNERT 1983) that were transferred to and assembled on target membranes. Similar analyses were carried out by HENKART et al. (1985) using a cytolytic rat tumor cell line of large granular morphology. These results led to the concept that some aspects of lymphocyte-mediated cytolysis are quite similar to the mechanism of complement-mediated cytolysis (for review, see PODACK 1986; PODACK and TSCHOPP 1984). Because the effector molecule of cytotoxic lymphocytes seemed to perforate the target membrane, it was designated "perforin 1" or "P1" (DENNERT and PODACK 1983). The assembly of P1 into transmembrane tubules resembles the formation of complement membrane lesions by polymerization of C9 (TSCHOPP et al. 1982; PODACK and TSCHOPP 1982b). The membrane lesions formed by effector lymphocytes were therefore designated "poly perforin" or "poly P1."

Morphological studies of cytotoxic thymus-dependent lymphocyte (CTL) or NK-target interaction suggested that the cytoplasmic granules con-

Department of Microbiology and Immunology, University of Miami School of Medicine, Miami, FL 33101, USA

Current Topics in Microbiology and Immunology, Vol. 140
© Springer-Verlag Berlin · Heidelberg 1988

tained in cytotoxic effector lymphocytes might be involved in effecting lymphocyte-mediated cytolysis. This concept received strong support by the isolation of these granules (PODACK and KONIGSBERG 1984; MILLARD et al. 1984; MASSON et al. 1985; YOUNG et al. 1986c) and the demonstration that the isolated granules are endowed with extraordinarily strong cytotoxicity when mixed with target cells in the presence of Ca. The target cells lysed by isolated granules showed the same poly P1 lesions observed previously when intact effector cells were used for the lysis of target cells.

Taken together, these studies resulted in the new hypothesis that target cell lysis by effector lymphocytes is mediated by the vectorial secretion of granules in a contact-dependent reaction onto the surface of the target cells. The formation of transmembrane channels by poly P1, in association with other factors causing target DNA degradation (RUSSELL et al. 1982; DUKE et al. 1983), may thus constitute the lethal hit responsible for the slow demise of the target cell.

This concept was fertile in that it stimulated the investigation of the composition of cytolytic granules and led to the discovery of groups of proteases whose interesting structure and function are described elsewhere in this book. Since other factors comprising granules are still under investigation, the list of components contributing to lymphocyte-mediated cytolysis via vectorial granule secretion is still growing.

2 The Poly Perforin Complex

The poly P1 complex is a tubular homopolymeric complex consisting of approximately twenty P1-protomers. The internal diameter of the poly P1 tubule measures 16 nm and its length is also 16 nm. Towards the membrane, the P1 subunits bear an externally hydrophobic face of approximately 4 nm in length that enables the complex to be stably integrated in target membranes. The internal surface of the poly P1 tubule is hydrophilic and thus creates a large (16 nm) transmembrane channel in the target membrane. These aspects of poly P1 are quite similar to those of poly C9, except that the internal diameter of poly C9 is only 10 nm.

Poly P1 can exist as a circular polymer (poly $P1_{20}$) or as a complex in which the tubule is not closed. The latter is formed by oligomers with varying protomer numbers (range 2–18 subunits). These open tubular complexes also effect transmembrane channels, albeit of smaller functional diameter, varying in size from approximately 2–14 nm (PODACK and TSCHOPP 1982b; YOUNG et al. 1986d). These transmembrane pores in all likelihood are partly walled by protein (oligo P1) and by rearranged (micellar?) lipid.

3 Isolation and Properties of Perforin

Using purified cytolytic granules as starting material, monomeric P1 has been isolated by several groups (MASSON and TSCHOPP 1985; HENKART et al. 1985;

PODACK et al. 1985; YOUNG et al. 1986c) from mouse and rat lymphocytes. Subsequently, it was also purified from human large granular lymphocytes (ZALMAN et al. 1986). Murine P1 is a 70 K–75 K protein of acidic isoelectric point. Purified P1, in the presence of Ca ions, lyses erythrocytes and nucleated target cells through polymerization and formation of transmembrane lesions in the target membrane. Although not yet studied in detail, it is assumed that the polymerization process of P1 resembles that of C9 and entails the Ca-dependent unfolding of the monomer from a hydrophilic globular molecule to an elongated amphiphilic protomer of the poly P1 complex. This process has to occur in close proximity to the target membrane to allow the simultaneous polymerization and insertion of P1 protomers into the lipid bilayer. If P1 polymerization occurs in the fluid phase, subsequent insertion of the amphiphilic poly P1 complex does not occur, presumably owing to thermodynamic barriers resulting from the necessity to displace laterally large numbers of phospholipid molecules. The insertional energy derived from the polymerization-unfolding process is thus dissipated in the fluid phase.

These properties of P1 explain why it cannot act from the fluid phase under in vivo conditions. They also explain its inactivation by preincubation of the cytolytic granules or of purified P1 in the presence of Ca (PODACK et al. 1985). Release of P1 into a Ca-containing environment results in rapid P1 polymerization and, as mentioned above, the poly P1 complex formed is incapable of inserting into membranes and hence causing cytolysis. P1 is also inhibited by serum factors such as lipoproteins and S protein and may be by others. Lipoproteins may compete with membranes for insertion of P1 whereas S protein, as shown for C5b-9 of complement (PODACK et al. 1984), may interfere with polymerization of P1.

Target cell lysis thus occurs only under stringent conditions as the exclusion of plasma proteins is required at the site at which granules are secreted within the contact area of NK-target conjugates. Moreover, this site must control the flux of Ca ions to prevent premature P1 polymerization, yet allow Ca entry when the polymerization of P1 takes place on the target membrane. How this is accomplished is poorly understood, although the observed wave of Ca flux within the NK cells upon target conjugation from distal to proximal areas of the effector cell clearly supports a strict regulation of Ca fluxes during target cell lysis.

4 The Structure of Perforin

The previous discussion emphasized similarities between complement component C9 and P1 in functional and structural terms. A homology of these two proteins and of C8, C7, and C6 is further supported by immunological cross-reactivities between the four terminal complement proteins and P1 (PODACK 1987; TSCHOPP et al. 1986; YOUNG et al. 1986a). This cross-reactivity and studies on the C5b-9 complex (PODACK et al. 1984; PODACK 1984) led to the concept that components C6, C7, C8, C9, and P1 are members of a phylogenetically related, pore-forming protein family, designated the perforin family. According to this hypothesis, C9 and P1 arose by gene duplication from an ancestor gene. P1 remained cell associated, whereas C9 became part of the secreted humoral immune system and further gave rise to $C8\alpha$, $C8\beta$, C7, and C6.

This concept has now been confirmed by primary structure analysis of all members of this family except C6, which is still outstanding (DiScipio et al. 1984, 1988; Haefliger et al. 1987; Howard et al. 1987; Rao et al. 1987). The structure of murine P1 is being elucidated by cDNA sequencing in our laboratory and, although not yet completed, clearly supports its homology to the complement proteins (Lowrey et al. 1987). We have aligned the sequence of P1 with C9, beginning from amino acid 120 of C9 to the C-terminus of C9. The computer-assisted alignment determined approximately 22% amino acid identity. Structural features believed to be of importance in C9 are conserved in the P1 sequence. These include homology in the putative membrane-binding site and conservation of the EGF-type, cysteine-rich domain located close to the C-terminus of C9. The length of the coding region of P1 contains a C-terminal extension of 140 amino acids not present in C9. We speculate that this C-terminal extension of P1 is related to its increased insertional efficiency when compared with C9.

5   Human Perforin

Studies on human P1, also designated C9-related protein (Zalman et al. 1986), showed similarities and discrepancies to murine P1. They are similar in molecular weight, cross-reactivity with anti-C9, and morphology of the poly P1 complex. In functional assays a difference was found, as human P1 exhibits only low or undetectable hemolytic activity (Lowrey et al. 1988). Why human P1 and granules from human large granular lymphocytes lack rapid hemolytic activity while containing factors mediating slow lysis of nucleated cells remains to be explained. Structurally, human P1, as far as it has yet been investigated, is homologous to murine P1. Amino acid identity of approximately 65% was seen in a partial sequence which also contains the C-terminal extension of murine P1 (M. Lichtenheld et al., Nature, in press).

6   Perforin-mRNA Expression

To date, a number of CTL and NK-like murine clones, as well as activated cytolytic lymphocyte populations, have been analyzed. Radiolabeled murine P1-cDNA probes hybridize with a single transcript of 2.9 kb in Northern blot analysis of cytotoxic cells but not with RNA derived from noncytotoxic lymphocytes or other cells and cell lines. The pattern of P1-mRNA expression is consistent with a role of P1 in the lymphocyte-mediated cytotoxicity of both CD4 and CD8 killer lymphocytes. In murine and human cytotoxic lymphocytes a

Table 1. Results of Northern blot experiments

P1-mRNA positive cells	P1-mRNA negative cells
1. Cloned CTL; class I MHC restricted: a) Virus (LCMV) specific syngeneic b) Hapten specific syngeneic c) Allogeneic	Monocytes Bone marrow derived macrophages B cells (unstimulated) B cells (stimulated, LPS-blasts) T cells (unstimulated) T lymphomas B lymphomas Fibroblasts
2. Cloned CTL; class II MHC restricted: a) Ovalbumin specific syngeneic (L3T4 pos.)	
3. Cloned CTL; non-MHC-restricted: a) Promiscuous killers (non-MHC-restricted)	
4. Cell populations: a) Concanavalin A stimulated spleen cells (day 3 and later) b) IL2 activated spleen cells (LAK cells) c) Mixed lymphocyte culture across class I MHC ($>$ day 3) d) Mixed lymphocyte culture across class II MHC ($>$ day 3) e) Syngeneic lymphocyte culture with virus infected (LCMV, vaccinia) syngeneic cells f) Stimulation of spleen cells with anti-T3	

single mRNA of identical size was found in either species. The murine cell line used was a CTL clone that has NK-like killing specificity (HY3 Ag3; ACHA-ORBEA et al. 1983), whereas the human RNA was obtained from human peripheral blood leukocytes (PBL) cultured for 3 weeks in 1000 U/ml rIL2 (LAK cells). Table 1   summarizes the results of Northern blot experiments with a variety of murine cloned CTL and mixed lymphocyte reactions. The important features emerging from this analysis are as follows:

1. In all situations in which cytotoxic activity is detectable, P1-mRNA is present; this includes in vivo-generated, virus-specific CTL (data not shown).
2. P1-mRNA is expressed both by MHC-restricted and non-MHC-restricted cytotoxic lymphocytes.
3. CD4-positive, class II MHC-restricted, so-called helper-killer cells are positive for P1-mRNA upon antigen stimulation. When mixed lymphocyte reactions across class II MHC barriers alone are set up, CD4 positive killer cells develop which contain P1-mRNA of characteristic size.
4. The induction period of P1-mRNA in precursor CTL requires 3 days and precedes cytotoxicity by approximately 12 h.
5. P1-mRNA is induced in precursor effector T cells in the absence of antigen by concanavalin A or high doses of rIL2. Such induction is not found in B cells or macrophages even after LPS stimulation.
6. In effector cells higher levels of P1-mRNA are induced by treatment with Ca-ionophores and phorbolesters.
7. P1-mRNA, in contrast to lymphokine messages, is not superinducible by cycloheximide.

Although these studies are consistent with the hypothesis that P1 is important in the cytolytic event mediated by killer lymphocytes, further experiments are necessary to determine whether P1 is essential for lymphocyte-mediated cytolysis in vivo and in vitro.

Acknowledgments. These studies were supported by funds from the American Cancer Society IM-369A, and USPHS grants A1-21999 and CA-39201.

Note added in proof:
Since submission of this manuscript the sequence of murine and human perforin has been published: SHINKAI et al., Nature 324:525 (1988), LICHTENHELD et al., Nature, in press (1988)

References

Acha-Orbea H, Grosscurth P, Lang R, Stitz L, Hengartner H (1983) Characterization of cloned cytotoxic lymphocytes with NK-like activity. J Immunol 130:2952–2959

Dennert G, Podack ER (1983) Cytolysis by H2-specific T killer cells: assembly of tubular complexes on target membranes. J Exp Med 157:1483–1495

Di Scipio RG, Gehring MR, Podack ER, Kan CC, Hugli TE, Fey GH (1984) Nucleotide sequence of cDNA and derived amino acid sequence of human complement component C9. Proc Natl Acad Sci USA 81:7298–7302

Di Scipio, RG, Chakravati, DN, Muller-Eberhard HJ, Fey GH (1988) The structure of human complement component C7 and the C5b-7 complex. J Biol Chem 263:549–555

Dourmashkin RR, Deteix P, Simone, CB, Henkart PA (1980) Electron microscopic demonstration of lesions on target cell membranes associated with antibody-dependent cytotoxicity. Clin Exp Immunol 43:554

Duke RC, Chervenak R, Cohen JJ (1983) Endogenous endonuclease-induced DNA fragmentation: an early event in cell-mediated cytolysis. Proc Natl Acad Sci USA 80:6361

Haefliger JA, Tschopp J, Nardelli D, Wahli W, Kocher HP, Stanley KK (1987) Complementary DNA cloning of complement C8β and its sequence homology to C9. Biochemistry 26:3551–3554

Henkart PA, Millard P, Yue C, Frederickse P, Blumenthal R, Bluestone J, Reynolds CW, Henkart MP (1985) Biochemical and functional properties of LGL and cytoplasmic granules. In: Henkart, Mertz (eds) Mechanism of cell mediated cytotoxicity II. Plenum, New York, p 85

Howard OMZ, Rao AG, Sodetz JM (1987) Complementary DNA and derived amino acid sequence of the b-subunit of human complement protein C8: identification of a close structural and ancestral relationship to the a-subunit and C9. Biochemistry 26:3565–3573

Lowrey DM, Rupp F, Aebischer T, Grey P, Hengartner H, Podack ER (1987) Primary sequence homology between the effector molecules that mediate complement and lymphocyte cytotoxicity. Ann Inst Pasteur Immunol 318:296–300

Lowrey DM, Hameed A, Lichtenheld M, Podack ER (1988) Isolation and characterization of cytotoxic granules from human lymphokine-(IL-2) activated Killer cells. Cancer Res (in press) Masson D, Tschopp J (1985) Isolation of a lytic pore forming protein (perforin) from cytolytic T lymphocytes. J Biol Chem 260:9069–0973

Masson D, Corthesy P, Nabholz M, Tschopp J (1985) Appearance of cytolytic granules upon induction of cytolytic activity in CTL-hybrids. EMBO J 4:2533–2538

Millard PJ, Henkart MP, Reynolds CW, Henkart PA (1984) Purification and properties of cytoplasmic granules from cytotoxic rat LGL tumors. J Immunol 132:3197

Podack ER (1984) Molecular composition of the tubular structure of the membrane attack complex of complement. J Biol Chem 259:8641–8642

Podack ER (1986) Molecular mechanism of cytolysis by complement and by cytolytic lymphocytes. J Cell Biochem 30:133–170

Podack ER (1987) Perforins: a family of pore forming proteins in immune cytolysis. In: *Membrane mediated cytoxocity.* Liss, New York, pp 339–352

Podack ER, Dennert G (1983) Assembly of two types of tubules with putative cytolytic function by cloned natural killer cells. Nature 302:442

Podack ER, Konigsberg PJ (1984) Cytolytic T cell granules. Isolation, biochemical and functional characterization. J Exp Med 160:695

Podack ER, Tschopp J (1982a) Circular polymerization of the ninth component of complement. J Biol Chem 257:15204–15212

Podack ER, Tschopp J (1982b) Polymerization of the ninth component of complement (C9): formation of poly C9 with a tubular ultrastructure resembling the membrane attack complex of complement. Proc Natl Acad Sci USA 79:574–578

Podack ER, Tschopp J (1984) Membrane attack by complement. Mol Immunol 21:589–603

Podack ER, Preissner K, Muller-Eberhard HJ (1984) Inhibition of C9 polymerization within the C5b-9 complex of complement by S-protein. Acta Pathol Microbiol Immunol Scand [C] [Suppl] 284:92:89–96

Podack ER, Young JDE, Cohn ZA (1985) Isolation and biochemical and functional characterization of perforin 1 from cytolytic T cell granules. Proc Natl Acad Sci USA 82:8629–8633

Rao AG, Howard OMZ, Ng SC, Whitehead AS, Colten HR, Sodetz JM (1987) Complementary DNA and derived amino acid sequence of the α-subunit of human complement protein C8: evidence for the existence of a separate subunit mRNA. Biochemistry 26:3556–3564

Russell JH, Masakowski V, Rucinsky T, Phillips G (1982) Mechanisms of immune lysis. III. Characterization of the nature and kinetics of the cytotoxic T lymphocyte-induced nuclear lesion in the target. J Immunol 128:2087

Tschopp J, Muller-Eberhard MJ, Podack ER (1982) Formation of transmembrane tubules by spontaneous polymerization of the hydrophilic complement protein C9. Nature 298:534–538

Tschopp J, Masson D, Stanley KK (1986) Structural/functional similarity between proteins involved in complement and cytotoxic T-lymphocyte mediated cytolysis. Nature 322:831–834

Young JDE, Cohn AZ, Podack ER (1986a) The ninth component of complement and the pore forming protein (perforin 1) from cytotoxic T-cells: structural, immunological and functional similarities. Science 233:184–190

Young JDE, Hengartner H, Podack ER, Cohn ZA (1986b) Purification and characterization of a cytolytic pore forming protein from granules of cloned lymphocytes with natural killer activity. Cell 44:849–859

Young JDE, Nathan CF, Podack ER, Palladino MA, Cohn ZA (1986c) Functional channel formation associated with cytotoxic T-cell granules. Proc Natl Acad Sci USA 83:150–154

Young JDE, Podack ER, Cohn ZA (1986d) Properties of a purified pore forming protein isolated from H2 restricted cytotoxic T-cell granules. J Exp Med 164:144–155

Zalman LS, Brothers MA, Chin F, Muller-Eberhard HJ (1986) Mechanism of cytotoxicity of human LGL: relationship of the cytotoxic lymphocyte protein to the ninth component of human complement. Proc Natl Acad Sci USA 83:5262–5266

Structure and Function of C8 in the Membrane Attack Sequence of Complement

J.M. SODETZ

1   Introduction 19
2   Functional Organization of C8 20
2.1 C8β 21
2.2 C8α 22
2.3 C8γ 23
3   Structure of C8 2
3.1 Genetic Basis 23
3.2 C8α 23
3.3 C8β 25
3.4 C8γ 26
4   Structural Similarities Between α, β, and C9 and Functional Implications 27
5   Synthesis 28
6   Conclusion 29
References 29

1 Introduction

Complement-mediated cell lysis occurs as a result of interactions between complement proteins C5b, C6, C7, C8, and C9 to produce the membrane attack complex C5b-9 (MÜLLER-EBERHARD 1986):

$$C5b \xrightarrow{C6} C5b\text{-}6 \xrightarrow{C7} C5b\text{-}7 \xrightarrow{C8} C5b\text{-}8 \xrightarrow{nC9} C5b\text{-}9$$

Assembly of C5b-9 begins with proteolytic conversion of C5 to C5b by the C5 convertases formed as a consequence of complement activation. Development of a transient binding site for C6 leads to formation of a stable C5b-6 dimer. Subsequent binding of C7 and formation of C5b-7 coincides with the expression of a high-affinity lipid-binding site that mediates a strong but noncovalent interaction between the nascent complex and target membranes. Binding of C8 yields the tetramolecular C5b-8 complex. Although capable of slowly lysing erythrocytes and some nucleated cells, C5b-8 functions primarily as a

Department of Chemistry and School of Medicine, University of South Carolina, Columbia, SC 29208, USA

Current Topics in Microbiology and Immunology, Vol. 140
© Springer-Verlag Berlin · Heidelberg 1988

receptor for C9 and thereby mediates formation of the more lytically effective C5b-9 complex. The number of C9 molecules per complex differs depending on C9 input and conditions of formation. The ultrastructure varies accordingly from what are functional lesions with one or a few C9s to highly organized porelike structures formed by polymerization of as many as 16 C9s per C5b-8. Facts and controversies about the function of C9 and the stoichiometry, structure, and mechanism of action of C5b-9 are summarized in other reports (PODACK 1986; MÜLLER-EBERHARD 1986; ESSER 1987; STANLEY, this volume). This review focuses strictly on C8 and its properties and structure-function relationships pertinent to its role in C5b-9 formation and function.

In several respects, assembly of C5b-9 is a unique biological process. It occurs by a strictly nonenzymatic mechanism, and aside from C5, no proteolytic cleavages occur in the constituent proteins. Likewise, lipids in the target membrane are not enzymatically degraded but instead undergo a disruptive rearrangement as a consequence of direct interaction with C5b-9. Also interesting is the ability of these five proteins to circulate independently in serum, yet associate in a highly specific sequence as a consequence of a single proteolytic cleavage in C5. This means that the interaction between components must induce an appropriate change in specificity such that the next component in the sequence can be recognized. Whether specificity is determined by large, conformationally defined domains or specific sequences on each constituent remains unknown. It is also noteworthy that binding interactions are noncovalent yet still occur with remarkably high affinity. Dissociation can only be accomplished by solubilizing membranes and denaturing the complexes. Perhaps most intriguing is that constituents of C5b-9 behave as hydrophilic proteins as they exist independently in serum, but when combined they form an amphiphilic complex capable of disrupting membranes. Hence, they must contain well-defined structural domains that mediate an association with lipid. Accessibility of these domains is most likely controlled by conformational changes during C5b-9 formation.

2   Functional Organization of C8

Among components of C5b-9, C8 has the most complex and unusual subunit structure. The human protein has a M_r of 151000 and contains an α (64000), β (64000), and γ (22000) subunit (KOLB and MÜLLER-EBERHARD 1976; STECKEL et al. 1980). These are arranged as a disulfide-linked α-γ dimer that is noncovalently associated with β. Evidence that C8 contains well-defined functional domains first emerged from efforts to purify these subunits (STECKEL et al. 1980). After purification in the presence of sodium dodecyl sulfate and removal of detergent, α-γ and β were found to recombine fully in dilute solution when mixed in equimolar ratios. Recombined C8 exhibited normal hemolytic activity and assumed a conformation similar to native C8 (MONAHAN and SODETZ 1980). Thus, it was concluded that domain(s) which mediate α-γ and β association are either stable to denaturation or can fully renature after exposure to detergent. This suggested that other intrinsic functional characteristics might be retained

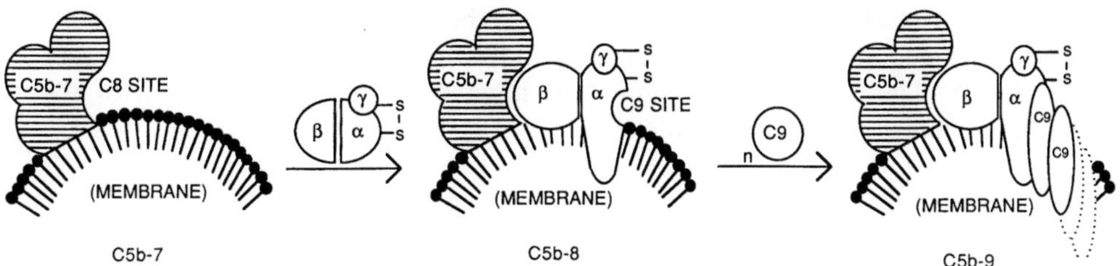

Fig. 1. Formation of C5b-8 and C5b-9 and topology of C8. The arrangement of C8 subunits is based on results described in the text. The transmembrane orientation of polymeric C9 reflects its ability to form channels alone or in C5b-9

by the isolated subunits and prompted a series of studies aimed at identifying functional domains in each subunit. From these studies, a model evolved for the topographical arrangement of C8 within C5b-8 and C5b-9 (Fig. 1).

2.1 C8 β

It is most appropriate to describe functional domains on β first since this subunit mediates C8 incorporation into the nascent C5b-9 complex (Fig. 1). Binding studies using purified subunits and C5b-7 on erythrocyte membranes showed that β alone binds with an affinity comparable to intact C8 (MONAHAN and SODETZ 1981). Whether binding is mediated through a conformationally defined domain on β or involves a receptor-ligand type interaction based on a specific sequence remains to be determined. Evidence does suggest that at least one essential tyrosine is involved (BRICKNER et al. 1985). More recent results indicate that binding is mediated through association with C5b in C5b-7, thus supporting the existence of a β-binding site on C5b and a key role for this protein in C5b-8 formation (STEWART et al. 1987). Interestingly, the α-γ subunit has no affinity for C5b-7 and therefore no direct role in C8 binding. However, it is required for C5b-9 formation since C5b-7(β) does not bind C9.

A second functional domain on β mediates its interaction with α-γ. This domain was identified in experiments using α and γ that were purified after limited reduction and alkylation of α-γ. Only α could associate with β to yield a stable α·β dimer referred to as C8′ (BRICKNER and SODETZ 1984). This dimer is functionally equivalent to native C8 with regard to binding C5b-7, mediating C9 incorporation and promoting cell lysis. Consequently, it was concluded that γ is not essential for C8 cytolytic activity.

A third functional domain on β can be broadly characterized as one or more segments that interact directly with the target membrane. Experimental support for this comes from photolabeling studies using photosensitive, membrane-restricted probes in synthetic lipid vesicles (HU et al. 1981; PODACK et al. 1981) and erythrocyte membranes (STECKEL et al. 1983). The β subunit was found to be one of several constituents of C5b-8 and C5b-9 labeled by these probes and therefore was assumed to be in direct contact with the membrane bilayer. One study that compared relative labeling of all three C8 subunits found β to be only moderately labeled in both C5b-8 and C5b-9 (STECKEL et al. 1983). Therefore, it is assumed to have only limited contact with the membrane surface in these complexes.

2.2 C8α

Four distinct functional domains have been identified on α (Fig. 1). One mediates α-γ association with β as demonstrated in the above experiments using purified α and β. A second domain appears to have a direct role in the lytic function of C5b-9. Studies using membrane-restricted probes revealed α to be the predominant component labeled within C5b-8 (STECKEL et al. 1983). Both α and C9 are also heavily labeled in C5b-9. This supports earlier conclusions that C9 has a major role in membrane lysis but further suggests that α also participates through direct insertion into the lipid bilayer.

A third functional domain on α consists of a single binding site for C9. Evidence for this site first came from the observation that C8 and C9 could associate in solution (KOLB et al. 1973; PODACK et al. 1982). Subsequent studies with purified subunits revealed a high affinity between α and C9, thus establishing that C8-C9 interactions involve a specific subunit (STEWART and SODETZ 1985). These same experiments showed that C5 could simultaneously associate with this dimer to yield a C5-C8-C9 complex in solution. These findings support a mechanism for C5b-9 formation in which C8 binds through association of its β subunit with C5b in C5b-7, after which C9 can associate through direct interaction with α. Conformational changes induced in the first C9 bound must then promote C9-C9 interactions leading to formation of the C9 polymeric structure found in fully formed C5b-9. This is consistent with the presumed ultrastructure of C5b-9 on lysed membranes (PODACK 1984), in which β is associated with C5b while C6, C7, α-γ, and C9 form a detergent-resistent copolymer.

A fourth domain on α is involved in direct interaction with γ. Recent studies found that α and γ retain a remarkably high affinity for each other after selective cleavage of the interchain disulfide and purification of each subunit (BRICKNER and SODETZ 1985). This could only occur if α has a specific binding site for γ. The significance of this interaction probably relates to the fact that unlike disulfide-linked subunits that have single chain precursors, α and γ are synthesized independently and must undergo intracellular association prior to disulfide bond formation (NG et al. 1987; NG and SODETZ 1987).

The site of contact between α and γ is considered to be on the periphery of C5b-8 and C5b-9 (Fig. 1). There are two reasons for proposing this arrangement. One is the ability of γ to bind C5b-8′ and C5b-(8′)9, two analogues of normal complexes prepared by substituting C8′ for C8 (BRICKNER and SODETZ 1985). Binding can only occur if the site for interaction on α is accessible in C5b-8′ and remains so after incorporation of C9. Secondly, photolabeling experiments failed to detect any interaction of γ with the membrane surface, a finding consistent with its nonessential role in lysis and a peripheral location in C5b-8 and C5b-9 (STECKEL et al. 1983).

2.3 C8γ

Thus far, the only functional domain identified on γ is one that mediates binding to the γ-specific site on α. This site may have little significance in the function of mature C8 but is probably important in the biosynthesis of α-γ.

3 Structure of C8

3.1 Genetic Basis

The asymmetric arrangement of noncovalent and covalently associated subunits is unusual for a serum protein but consistent with evidence that C8 is assembled from different gene products. Support for this initially came from analyses of C8 protein polymorphisms in families (ALPER et al. 1983; RITTNER et al. 1984). Electrophoretic analysis of C8 under nonreducing conditions revealed that polymorphic patterns for α-γ and β segregate independently. It was later concluded that α-γ and β are encoded at separate but closely linked genetic loci on chromosome 1 (ROGDE et al. 1986). This conclusion was supported by the fact that in human C8 deficiencies, structural and functional abnormalities are associated with α-γ or β but not with both subunits (TEDESCO et al. 1983). Implicit in these findings were the existence of separate genes for α-γ and β and the likelihood that α-γ would be synthesized in single-chain precursor form.

Recent isolation of cDNA clones for α, β, and γ from a human liver cDNA library has suggested otherwise (RAO et al. 1987; HOWARD et al. 1987; NG et al. 1987). All three cDNAs have 5′ and 3′ sequences that are consistent with separate and distinct mRNAs for each, e.g. initiation Met, poly A sequences. Analysis of RNA from the human hepatoma cell line HepG2 and baboon liver confirmed the presence of separate mRNAs. These results and the lack of nucleotide sequence homology amongst their respective cDNAs indicate that α, β, and γ are encoded in not two (α-γ and β) but three (α, β, and γ) separate genes.

This conclusion is compatible with genetic data on C8 polymorphisms if one realizes that those results were obtained by electrophoretic analysis performed under nonreducing conditions. Consequently, a distinction between α and γ polymorphisms could not be made. In one study that examined C8 under reducing conditions, it was found that polymorphisms in α-γ are in fact attributable to only α (ROGDE et al. 1985). This is significant because instead of two separate loci for α-γ and β, an equally valid explanation for nonreduced electrophoretic patterns is the existence of three loci with detectable allelic variation in α and β but not γ.

3.2 C8α

The amino acid sequence of the human α subunit was derived by analysis of a 2.4-kb cDNA clone (RAO et al. 1987). This subunit is synthesized with a leader sequence (30 residues) consisting of an apparent signal peptide and pro-

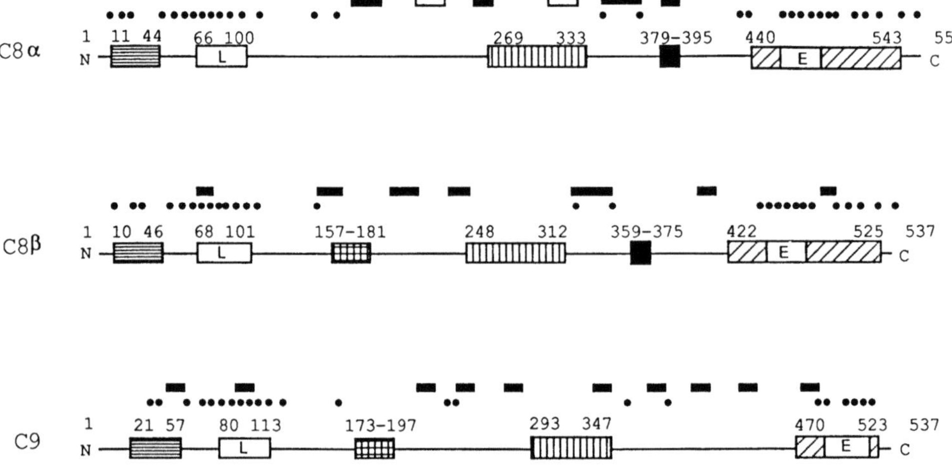

Fig. 2. Summary of structural similarities between C8α, C8β, and C9. Segments of C8α, C8β, and C9 related by sequence homology are identified by residue numbers and common markings. All segments exhibit ≥39% identity and ≥54% homology if conserved substitutions are included. Segments containing the low density lipoprotein receptor homology are identified by *L*, and those with epidermal growth factor precursor homology by *E*. Cysteine residues are identified by *solid circles*. *Solid bars* above each protein identify predicted membrane surface-seeking segments while *open bars* identify predicted transmembrane segments. Data for C8α is from Rao et al. (1987) and data for C8β is from Howard et al. (1987). For C9, the sequence (Di Scipio et al. 1984), identification of LDL and EGFP domains (Stanley et al. 1985), and the location of predicted membrane surface-seeking segments (Shiver et al. 1986) were reported by others. It is noted that the number of cysteines shown here for C9 differs by one from that reported by others (Stanley et al. 1985). This figure is a revision of one in Howard et al. (1987)

peptide. This is followed by the sequence of 553 residues found in mature α. The calculated M_r 61 460 agrees well with the M_r 64 000 reported for the glycosylated subunit (Steckel et al. 1980). Carbohydrate analyses indicate 1-2 asparagine and no *O*-linked carbohydrate chains. RNA blot analysis revealed a message size of 2.5 kb in HepG2 cells and baboon liver.

There are several noteworthy features of the amino acid sequence (Fig. 2). The N- and C-termini are both cysteine rich while the central region is relatively free of cysteines. The N-terminus exhibits strong homology to the 40-residue repeat sequence found in the low density lipoprotein (LDL) receptor. This homology includes conserved cysteines and a clustering of negatively charged residues. The C-terminus exhibits homology to a highly conserved segment found in epidermal growth factor precursor (EGFP) and several other proteins including urokinase, blood coagulation factors FIX and FX, and tissue plasminogen activator.

Hydropathic analysis reveals no extended hydrophobic segments but the predictive method of Eisenberg et al. (1984) identified several segments with the potential for interacting with membranes. Four satisfy the criteria for membrane surface-seeking segments, and two appear typical of α-helical transmembrane segments that interact cooperatively in pairs or multimers in channel-forming proteins. Interestingly, the latter two segments must assume an α-helical conformation to satisfy the criteria for transmembrane domains. However, these are predicted to be β-sheet structures if α is considered to be a typical globular protein. This means these segments must undergo a conformational change from β-sheet to α-helix during C8 binding to C5b-7 in order to become transmembrane. Such a change may explain why C8 alone has no affinity for membranes yet can insert into the bilayer after incorporation into C5b-8.

Location of both candidate transmembrane segments occurs in the cysteine-free central region of α. Intrinsic flexibility is therefore possible and could facilitate conformational changes needed to expose these domains during C8 binding. Also noteworthy is the absence of cysteines between the two segments. If they actually span the bilayer of a target membrane rather than simply penetrate, then an intervening segment of ~ 69 residues must appear on the cytoplasmic side. The absence of cysteines in this region would permit a linearized conformation for translocation across the membrane. Experimental support for a transmembrane orientation includes one study showing that within C5b-8 and C5b-9, C8 can be cross-linked from the cytoplasmic side of erythrocyte ghosts (WHITLOW et al. 1985). Photolabeling results also indicate that direct interaction between α and the bilayer is likely (STECKEL et al. 1983).

3.3 C8β

The amino acid sequence of human β was also derived from cDNA sequencing (HOWARD et al. 1987). Characterization of a 2.0-kb cDNA indicates that β has an unusually long leader sequence of 54 amino acids. This sequence has many features of a signal peptide but terminates with Arg, a residue rarely found at signal peptidase cleavage sites. This is followed by 537 residues corresponding to mature β. The calculated M_r 60951 agrees well with the 64000 reported earlier (STECKEL et al. 1980). Carbohydrate analysis revealed only 1-2 asparagine and no O-linked carbohydrate chains. RNA blot analysis identified mRNAs of 2.5 kb in HepG2 cells and 2.6 kb in baboon liver.

The amino acid sequence of β was reported simultaneously by this and another laboratory (HAEFLIGER et al. 1987). The published sequences agree with only two exceptions. One is position 63 where a single base substitution yields Arg instead of Gly, a probable consequence of characterizing different clones, i.e., a point mutation. The second is position 383–390 in the sequence of HOWARD et al. This segment not only differs in sequence but also contains one less amino acid than the corresponding sequence of HAEFLIGER et al. This laboratory has since reconciled differences in this region and confirmed that HAEFLIGER'S sequence is correct. Importantly, the error in the sequence of HOWARD et al. has no effect on conclusions regarding hydropathy, location of membrane-interacting domains, or homologies to other proteins.

Analysis of the β sequence reveals cysteine-rich N- and C-termini and a relatively cysteine-free central region (Fig. 2). Both the LDL receptor and EGFP consensus sequences are present, as are other segments of homology to α. Also present is the Arg-Gly-Asp sequence found at the cell recognition site of several cell adhesion proteins (RUOSLAHTI and PIERSCHBACHER 1987). The functional

significance of this sequence is unclear, but it may have a role in C8 binding
to C5b-7. Hydropathic analysis revealed no lengthy regions of hydrophobicity;
however, several membrane surface-seeking segments were identified. Interestingly, the prediction of surface-seeking rather than transmembrane segments
is consistent with photolabeling experiments showing that β interaction with
the target membrane is minimal (STECKEL et al. 1983).

3.4   C8γ

The sequence of human γ was derived from characterization of a 718-bp cDNA
clone (NG et al. 1987). An apparent signal peptide of 20 residues is followed
by 182 residues corresponding to a M_r 20329. Mature γ contains an N-terminal
pyroglutamyl residue and no carbohydrate. RNA blot analysis indicates a message size of 1.0 kb in baboon liver.

The sequence contains three cysteines, only one of which is probably linked
to α. There are no extended hydrophobic regions nor predicted membrane-
interacting segments. This is entirely consistent with the inability to detect γ
interaction with the membrane bilayer in photolabeling experiments (STECKEL
et al. 1983). It also supports the conclusion that γ is located in a hydrophilic
environment on the periphery of C5b-8 and C5b-9.

Since γ is not essential for C8 lytic activity, one can only speculate on
a functional role for this subunit. As noted recently by others (HUNT et al.
1987; DOOLITTLE 1988), γ belongs to a family of proteins that includes α_1-
microglobulin, protein HC (or human complex-forming glycoprotein), serum
retinol-binding protein, α_1-acid glycoprotein, β-lactoglobulin, and others. These
proteins have been termed "lipocalins" (PERVAIZ and BREW 1987) because of
their ability to bind lipophilic ligands, e.g., vitamin A, steroid hormones. Whether γ binds similar ligands is unknown, but one can speculate that if it does
have an affinity for lipophilic structures, it might function by interacting with
hydrophobic domains on α and thereby shield C8 from premature interactions
with membranes during posttranslational processing or while in the circulation.
This shielding would be relieved by conformational changes associated with
C8 binding to C5b-7.

There are other possible functions to consider. Among the lipocalins, protein
HC is reportedly an inhibitor of neutrophil chemotaxis (MENDEZ et al. 1986).
Thus, γ may have a related function as a regulator of the immune response
at the site of C5b-8 or C5b-9 formation. Another possible role for γ is that
it imparts a functional difference to two otherwise structurally similar subunits,
i.e., α and β. If so, this difference must be subtle because α alone can still
associate with β and function in cytolysis. Alternatively, it may be essential
for intracellular processing of α-γ or stability of C8 in the circulation. Most
intriguing is its possible role in regulating C8 activity and thereby protecting
host cells from lysis. Evidence suggests that interaction between γ and what
may be an ubiquitous cell-surface protein (homologous restriction factor) may
be an essential step in the mechanism by which homologous cells protect them-
selves from C5b-9 mediated lysis (HÄNSCH et al. 1986; ZALMAN et al. 1986).

Although yet to be characterized, this protein might contain a lipophilic moiety that mediates binding of γ. If so, it could explain the functional significance of the lipocalin-like structure of γ.

4 Structural Similarities Between α, β, and C9 and Functional Implications

Comparison of α, β, and human C9 reveals similarities that are indicative of a close ancestral relationship between all three proteins (Fig. 2). The overall sequence homology between α and β is 33% based on identity and 53% when conserved substitutions are included. Values are 24% and 46% for α and C9, and 26% and 47% for β and C9, respectively. These homologies include not only the LDL receptor and EGFP domains but other large regions as well. Each homologous region occurs at the same location in all three proteins, thus revealing a remarkable similarity in structural organization. This is further indicated by the similar number of amino acids, the concentration of cysteines at the N- and C-termini, and, for α and β, the nearly identical carbohydrate content.

Considering that these proteins are hydrophilic but can display amphiphilic characteristics, it is also significant that each contains segments capable of interacting with membranes. Most occur in a relatively cysteine-free region where conformational constraints are minimal. Such a design must have a purpose. As they exist independently in plasma, each protein must be refractory to membranes, yet still be able to expose membrane-interacting segments upon binding C5b-7 or C5b-8. A lack of intrachain disulfide bonds would allow flexibility and therefore exposure of such segments to be modulated by conformational changes, which in turn could be influenced by protein-protein interactions during assembly of each complex. Thus, one reason each protein may have this structural arrangement is to facilitate a function they have in common, a hydrophilic to amphiphilic transition and subsequent membrane association.

The presence of conserved domains in all three proteins may also provide a clue to the underlying mechanism of C5b-9 assembly. In solution, C8 and C9 can form a complex that is mediated by a single C9-binding site on α (STEWART and SODETZ 1985). Because α is simultaneously associated with β in C8, this complex must be physically arranged as β-α-C9. Furthermore, the ability of C9 to self-polymerize in solution or upon binding to C5b-8 suggests that a copolymer of β-α-C9-C9$_n$ could form within membrane-bound C5b-9 (Fig. 1). Considering this and similarities in α, β, and C9 structures, one can speculate that pairs of conserved domains might align to provide a repetitive structure leading to formation of such a copolymer. This might involve a network of electrostatic interactions between the negatively charged LDL receptor domain and positively charged segments elsewhere on each protein. The ionic strength dependency of α-β and α-C9 interactions in solution supports such a mechanism, as does the ability of positively charged peptides to inhibit self-polymerization of C9 (TSCHOPP et al. 1987).

Recent determination of the human C7 sequence revealed that it too is homologous to α, β, and C9 and contains LDL receptor and EGFP domains (DI SCIPIO et al. 1988). Thus, it may also participate in copolymer formation. If so, the report of a C6-C7-(α-γ)-C9n copolymer isolated from C5b-9 and the identification of a β-specific site on C5b argue against the possibility that C7 interacts solely with β. It is more likely that multiple, simultaneous interactions between components occur once C8 makes initial contact with C5b through its β subunit. This is supported by cross-linking results showing that within C5b-8, β is closely associated with C5b, C6, and C7 (STEWART et al. 1987).

On the basis of similarities in their structure and function, one must conclude that α, β, and C9 are members of a family of proteins that are capable of induced conformational changes leading to membrane interaction. The sequence of C7 suggests it also belongs to this family. Another likely member is perforin, the pore-forming protein released from cytotoxic lymphocytes. This protein facilitates lysis of target cells through self-polymerization and formation of pores that resemble C5b-9 formed on complement-lysed membranes. The perforin monomer is similar in size to C9, and like C9 it can be induced to self-polymerize by metal ions (PODACK et al., this volume). Immunological evidence also indicates that perforin and C9 have common antigenic determinants, at least one of which involves the cysteine-rich LDL receptor domain.

5 Synthesis

The primary site of C8 synthesis is the liver, but it is also produced by monocytes (HETLAND et al. 1986). Little is known about the intracellular processing and assembly of C8. A recent study using rat hepatocytes reported no evidence of a single-chain form of α-γ in the intracellular pool (NG and SODETZ 1987), a finding corroborated by cDNA analyses and identification of separate messages for α, β and γ in humans. There was also no detectable pool of free α or γ, indicating that these subunits are probably synthesized at similar rates, and that disulfide bond formation occurs cotranslationally or early in posttranslational processing. Similar rates suggest that expression of α and γ may be subject to common transcriptional and/or translational controls, a hypothesis that seems reasonable in view of their stoichiometric relationship. Early disulfide bond formation is also reasonable to expect and would be analogous to IgG or fibrinogen synthesis in which the component chains associate while at least one is still on the polysome. In the case of IgG, this occurs because of an intrinsic affinity between chains that persists even after reduction and alkylation. The intrinsic affinity between α and γ supports the likelihood that a similar noncovalent association occurs early in the processing of α-γ.

Biosynthesis studies also suggest that β may be regulated differently than α and γ. In rat hepatocytes, α-γ is synthesized significantly faster than β, and because they associate intracellularly in stoichiometric amounts, the faster synthetic rate results in secretion of excess α-γ. This was initially considered an artifact of cultured cells, but a recent report confirmed the presence of free

α-γ in normal human serum (DENSEN and NAUSEEF 1987). The functional significance of excess α-γ is unclear, but it may simply ensure that all intracellular β is converted to C8 prior to secretion. Residual α-γ would then be secreted independently.

6 Conclusion

Considerable progress has been made in our understanding of the structure-function relationships in C8. Identification of functional domains provides a firm basis for more refined studies of molecular interactions within C5b-9. Likewise, knowledge of the sequence has yielded a working hypothesis to explain the hydrophilic to amphiphilic transition by C8 and perhaps other constituents of C5b-9. Nevertheless, there are still important and intriguing questions to be answered. We must still determine why C8 evolved to serve as an intermediary between C5b-7 and C9 and why it is such a complex protein assembled from three different gene products. How is C8 assembled inside the cell? What is the function of the γ subunit? Is it possible that C8 has some function other than cytolysis, perhaps one that requires such an unusual quaternary structure? These and other questions will undoubtedly be answered in future studies of this interesting protein.

Acknowledgments. This effort was supported by NIH Grant AI16856 and Established Investigator Award 82-121 from the American Heart Association.

References

Alper CA, Marcus D, Raum D, Petersen BH, Spira TJ (1983) Genetic polymorphism in C8 β chains. J Clin Invest 72:1526–1531

Brickner A, Sodetz JM (1984) Function of subunits within the eighth component of human complement: selective removal of the γ chain reveals it has no direct role in cytolysis. Biochemistry 23:832–837

Brickner A, Sodetz JM (1985) Functional domains of the α-subunit of the eighth component of human complement: identification and characterization of a distinct binding site for the γ chain. Biochemistry 24:4603–4607

Brickner A, Lambert SJ, Sodetz JM (1985) Evidence that a single tyrosine in human C8 is essential for binding to C5b-7. Complement 2:13A

Densen P, Nauseef WM (1987) Biosynthesis of human C8. Complement 4:150A

Di Scipio RG, Gehring MR, Podack ER, Kan CC, Hugli TE, Fey GH (1984) Nucleotide sequence of cDNA and derived amino acid sequence of human complement component C9. Proc Natl Acad Sci USA 81:7298–7302

Di Scipio RG, Chakravarti DN, Müller-Eberhard HJ, Fey GH (1988) Structure of human C7 and the C5b-7 complex. J Biol Chem 263:549–560

Doolittle RF (1988) Redundancies in protein sequences. In: Fasman G (ed) Prediction of protein structure and the principles of protein conformation Plenum, New York (in press)

Eisenberg D, Schwarz E, Komaromy M, Wall R (1984) Analysis of membrane and surface protein sequences with the hydrophobic moment plot. J Mol Biol 179:125–142

Esser AF (1987) C9-mediated cytotoxicity and the function of poly (C9). In: Bonavida B, Collier RJ (eds) Membrane-mediated cytotoxicity. UCLA Symposia on Molecular and Cellular Biology, New Series, Vol. 45 Liss, New York, pp 411–422

Haefliger JA, Tschopp J, Nardelli D, Wahli W, Kocher HP, Tosi M, Stanley KK (1987) Complementary DNA cloning of complement C8 β and its sequence homology to C9. Biochemistry 26:3551–3556

Hänsch G, Schönermark S, Roelcke D (1986) The role of C8 binding protein in homologous species restriction of C-mediated lysis: the C8 bp interacts with the α-γ subunit of C8 and inhibits C9 polymerization. Fed Proc 45:247 A

Hetland G, Johnson E, Falk RJ, Eskeland T (1986) Synthesis of complement components C5, C6, C7, C8 and C9 in vitro by human monocytes and assembly of the terminal complement complex. Scand J Immunol 24:421–428

Howard OMZ, Rao AG, Sodetz JM (1987) Complementary DNA and derived amino acid sequence of the β subunit of human complement protein C8: Identification of a close structural and ancestral relationship to the α subunit and C9. Biochemistry 26:3565–3570

Hu VW, Esser AF, Podack ER, Wisnieski BJ (1981) Membrane attack mechanism of complement: photolabeling reveals insertion of terminal proteins into target membranes. J Immunol 127:380–386

Hunt LT, Elzanowski A, Barker WC (1987) The homology of complement factor C8 gamma chain and alpha-1-microglobulin. Biochem Biophys Res Commun 149:282–288

Kolb WP, Müller-Eberhard HJ (1976) The membrane attack mechanism of complement: the three polypeptide chain structure of the eighth (C8) component. J Exp Med 143:1131–1139

Kolb WP, Haxby JA, Arroyave CM, Müller-Eberhard HJ (1973) The membrane attack mechanism of complement. Reversible interactions among the five native components in free solution. J Exp Med 138:428–437

Mendez E, Fernandez-Luna JL, Grubb A, Cobian FL (1986) Human protein HC and its IgA complex are inhibitors of neutrophil chemotaxis. Proc Natl Acad Sci USA 83:1472–1475

Monahan JB, Sodetz JM (1980) Binding of the eighth component of human complement to the soluble cytolytic complex is mediated by its β-subunit. J Biol Chem 255:10579–10582

Monahan JB, Sodetz JM (1981) Role of the β-subunit in the interaction of the eighth component of human complement with the membrane-bound cytolytic complex. J Biol Chem 256:3258–3262

Müller-Eberhard HJ (1986) The membrane attack complex of complement. Annu Rev Immunol 4:503–528

Ng SC, Sodetz JM (1987) Biosynthesis of C8 by hepatocytes: differential expression and intracellular association of the α-γ and β subunits. J Immunol 139:3021–3027

Ng SC, Rao AG, Howard OMZ, Sodetz JM (1987) The eighth component of human complement (C8): evidence that it is an oligomeric serum protein assembled from products of three different genes. Biochemistry 26:5229–5233

Pervaiz S, Brew K (1987) Homology and structure-function correlations between α_1-acid glycoprotein and serum retinol-binding protein and its relatives. FASEB J 1:209–214

Podack ER (1984) Molecular composition of the tubular structure of the membrane attack complex of complement. J Biol Chem 259:8641–8647

Podack ER (1986) Molecular mechanisms of cytolysis by complement and by cytolytic lymphocytes. J Cell Biochem 30:133–170

Podack ER, Stoffel W, Esser AF, Müller-Eberhard HJ (1981) Membrane attack complex of complement: distribution of subunits between the hydrocarbon phase of target membranes and water. Proc Natl Acad Sci USA 78:4544–4548

Podack ER, Tschopp J, Müller-Eberhard HJ (1982) Molecular organization of C9 within the membrane attack complex of complement: induction of circular C9 polymerization by C5b-8. J Exp Med 156:268–282

Rao AG, Howard OMZ, Ng SC, Whitehead AS, Colten HR, Sodetz JM (1987) Complementary DNA and derived amino acid sequence of the α subunit of human complement protein C8: evidence for the existence of a separate α subunit mRNA. Biochemistry 26:3556–3564

Rittner C, Hargesheimer W, Mollenhauer E (1984) Population and formal genetics of the human C81 (α-γ) polymorphism. Hum Genet 67:166–169

Rogde S, Mevag B, Teisberg P, Gedde-Dahl T, Tedesco F, Olaisen B (1985) Genetic polymorphism of complement component C8. Hum Genet 70:211–216

Rogde S, Olaisen B, Gedde-Dahl T, Teisberg P (1986) The C8A and C8B loci are closely linked on chromosome 1. Ann Hum Genet 50:139–144

Ruoslahti E, Pierschbacher MD (1987) New perspectives in cell adhesion: RGD and integrins. Science 238:491–497

Shiver JW, Dankert JR, Donovan JJ, Esser AF (1986) The ninth component of human complement: functional activity of the b fragment. J Biol Chem 261:9629–9636

Stanley KK, Kocher H-P, Luzio JP, Jackson P, Tschopp J (1985) The sequence and topology of human complement component C9. EMBO J 4:375–381

Steckel EW, York RG, Monahan JB, Sodetz JM (1980) The eighth component of human complement. Purification and physicochemical characterization of its unusual subunit structure. J Biol Chem 255:11997–12005

Steckel EW, Welbaum BE, Sodetz JM (1983) Evidence of direct insertion of terminal complement proteins into cell membrane bilayers during cytolysis: labeling by a photosensitive membrane probe reveals a major role for the eighth and ninth components. J Biol Chem 258:4318–4324

Stewart JL, Sodetz JM (1985) Analysis of the specific association of the eighth and ninth components of human complement: identification of a direct role for the α subunit of C8. Biochemistry 24:4598–4602

Stewart JL, Kolb WP, Sodetz JM (1987) Evidence that C5b recognizes and mediates C8 incorporation into the cytolytic complex of complement. J Immunol 139:1960–1964

Tedesco F, Densen P, Villa MA, Petersen BH, Sirchia G (1983) Two types of dysfunctional eighth component of complement (C8) molecules in C8 deficiency in man: reconstitution of normal C8 from the mixture of two abnormal C8 molecules. J Clin Invest 71:183–191

Tschopp J, Masson D, Peitsch M (1987) Molecular mechanisms of C9 polymerization and its inhibition by S-protein. Complement 4:232 A

Whitlow MB, Ramm LE, Mayer MM (1985) Penetration of C8 and C9 in the C5b-9 complex across the erythrocyte membrane into the cytoplasmic space. J Biol Chem 260:998–1005

Zalman LS, Wood LM, Müller-Eberhard HJ (1986) Isolation of a human erythrocyte membrane protein capable of inhibiting expression of homologous complement transmembrane channels. Proc Natl Acad Sci USA 83:6975–6979

Granzymes: a Family of Serine Proteases in Granules of Cytolytic T Lymphocytes

D.E. Jenne and J. Tschopp

1 Introduction 33

2 Purification of CTL Granule Proteases 34

3 Substrates and Inhibitors of Granzymes 36

4 cDNA Cloning and Structural Features of Granzymes 38

5 Expression of Granzymes 43

6 Function of Granzymes 44

References 45

1 Introduction

Cellular serine proteases are most active at neutral, physiological pH and have been implicated in a variety of different processes such as cellular chemotaxis, protein turnover in tissues, endocytosis and exocytosis, or tumorigenesis (Neurath 1984). In addition, there is also considerable evidence that cellular proteases play an important role in cell-mediated cytotoxicity: T-cell killing can be inhibited by diisopropylfluorophosphate (DFP) or PMSF (Chang and Eisen 1980; Quan et al. 1982), suggesting DFP- or PMSF-inactivation of functionally important trypsin-like proteases. Antibody-dependent cell-mediated cytotoxicity is abolished by protease substrates such as acetyl tyrosine ester in a competitive manner, and by chloromethyl ketone derivatives of amino acids. Macromolecular antiproteases like $\alpha 1$-antitrypsin and $\alpha 1$-antichymotrypsin also suppress lysis when present in natural killer (NK) cell assays (Redelman and Hudig 1980; Hudig et al. 1981, 1984), further implicating the involvement of proteases in the cytotoxic event. While pretreatment of the effector cell with protease inhibitors has no effect on the lytic activity of NK cells, cytotoxicity is highly sensitive to the presence of inhibitors for a short period of time after the addition of the target cell (Lavie et al. 1985), suggesting that target cell binding triggers the exposure of enzymes to the external environment. A similar short period of time was observed when the sensitivity to microfilament inhibitors was tested (Lavie et al. 1985), indicating that a secretory process is involved in the release of the proteases (Quan et al. 1982). The most direct evidence, however, for the importance of proteases in the cytotoxic event comes from a report by

Institute of Biochemistry, University of Lausanne, CH-1066 Epalinges, Switzerland

HATCHER et al. (HATCHER et al. 1978), who demonstrated that a DFP-sensitive protease of T-cell origin was engaged in cytotoxicity against a human transitional cell carcinoma.

All these observations led to the proposal of an hypothesis in which initially cryptic proteases are released upon effector-target cell contact, enabling them to exert an as yet undefined role in cytotoxicity. However, none of these putative proteases has been isolated or characterized, mostly due to the difficulty in obtaining homogeneous cytolytic effector cells in quantities sufficient to allow the isolation of a reasonable amount of protein. This major difficulty was overcome when Il-2-dependent, cytolytic T-lymphocyte (CTL) clones became available (NABHOLZ and MacDONALD 1982). In 1985, several groups demonstrated that CTL contain dense cytoplasmic granules (PODACK and KÖNIGSBERG 1984; MILLARD et al. 1984; PODACK 1985, 1986; MASSON et al. 1985) which, in isolated form, were lytic towards a variety of tumor cell targets or red blood cells. Moreover, it was demonstrated that the contents of the granules were released upon conjugate formation of the CTL and the appropriate target cell (SCHMIDT et al. 1985; MacDERMOTT et al. 1985; GARCIA-SANZ et al. 1987; PASTERNACK et al. 1986; YOUNG et al. 1986a; TAKAYAMA et al. 1987). Subsequently, a lytic, pore-forming protein called perforin/cytolysin was isolated from the granules (MASSON and TSCHOPP 1985; PODACK et al. 1985; YOUNG et al. 1986b, c). This protein exhibits structural homology to complement component C9 (YOUNG et al. 1986d, e; TSCHOPP et al. 1986; see chapter 2 by PODACK et al., this volume). Perforin, however, is only one of several major constituents of the lytic granules (MASSON and TSCHOPP 1985; PODACK et al. 1985). Since CTL clones were shown to contain a high level of a protease which was very active on the synthetic substrate N-α-benzyloxycarbonyl-1-lysine thiobenzyl ester (BLT) (PASTERNACK and EISEN 1985), the possibility exists that one or several of these molecules is a protease(s).

Our group recently succeeded in characterizing all the major proteins found in granules of mouse CTL lines (MASSON and TSCHOPP 1987). They turned out to be highly homologous serine proteases, thereby supporting the notion that proteases may be implicated in CTL/NK cell-mediated cytolysis.

2 Purification of CTL Granule Proteases

Cytoplasmic granules are usually isolated by a Percoll density gradient (HENKART et al. 1984; PODACK and KÖNIGSBERG 1984; MASSON et al. 1985). High salt buffers are used to disrupt the granules. Analysis of the granule-associated proteins by sodium dodecylsulfate-polyacrylamide gel electrophoresis (SDS-PAGE) reveals at least six distinct protein bands ranging from 27 K–70 K (HENKART et al. 1984; PODACK and KÖNIGSBERG 1984; MASSON et al. 1985). Perforin is specifically removed from the protein mixture upon passage through a TSK 3000 column; for unknown reasons, the pore-forming protein is unspecifically retarded and elutes as pure protein after the total volume of the column (MASSON and TSCHOPP 1985). The remainder of the granule proteins is pooled

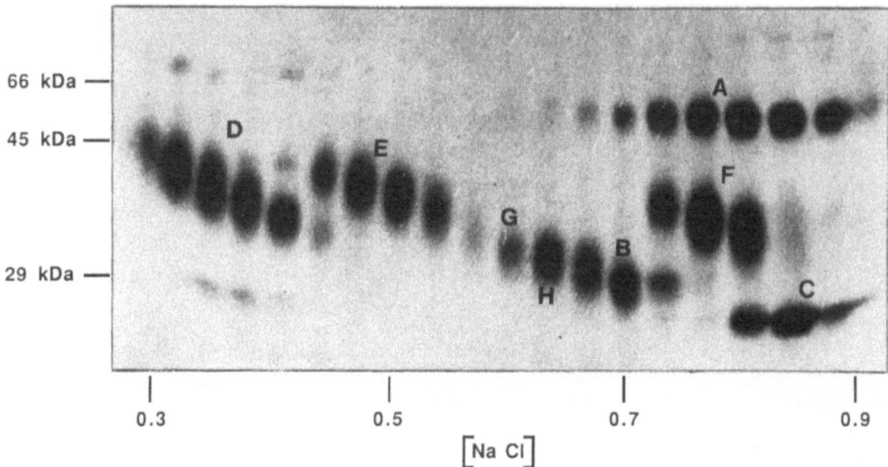

Fig. 1. Elution pattern of granzymes loaded onto a Mono S cation exchange column. Granule proteins of the CTL line B6.1, which had been depleted of perforin, were loaded onto a Mono S column. Subsequently, the proteins (granzymes A through G) were eluted by increasing the NaCl concentration

and loaded onto a Mono S strong cation exchange column (MASSON and TSCHOPP 1987). At 50 mM NaCl, pH 6.0, this type of column retains all major components and separates them well upon increasing the NaCl concentration. A typical elution pattern is shown in Fig. 1. Eight distinct protein bands are distinguishable upon SDS-PAGE of the various fractions. Since biochemical and cDNA sequence analysis has shown (see below) that the proteins are serine proteases, we propose the designation granzymes (granule-associated enzymes). This designation neither implies a tissue distribution nor a preference for a synthetic substrate as is the case with alternative names like T-cell-specific serine protease (SIMON et al. 1986), cytotoxic T-cell-specific protein (LOBE et al. 1986a, b), or BLT esterase (PASTERNACK and EISEN 1985), which have been proposed for two of these proteases.

The protein eluting first from the cation exchange column (at low salt concentration) is granzyme D. It forms a group of proteins with granzymes E and F (which elute at higher salt concentrations) and they are heterogenous in molecular size, ranging from 35 K–55 K. The fact that the larger molecules are eluted earlier than the smaller components suggests that the heterogeneity is due to different amounts of negatively charged carbohydrate moieties. Granzymes B, G, and H form a second related group which is not resolved by the cation exchanger. Their 20 N-terminal amino acid residues are identical, showing their extremely high similarity. Indeed, it cannot be excluded that granzymes B, G, and H represent differently glycosylated forms of the same molecule, thus accounting for their differences in molecular size (Table 1). Granzyme A elutes at 780 mM NaCl. It has a structure which is unique among serine proteases in that it forms a disulfide-linked homodimer, which explains the molecular weight shift from 60000 under nonreducing conditions, to 35000 under

Table 1. Serine protease family in granules of cytolytic T-lymphocytes

Serine protease	Corresponding cDNA clone[a]	Molecular mass (daltons)[b]	DFP-reactive	Substrates[c]	Elution from Mono S column (mM NaCl)	Other characteristics
Granzyme A	H factor	35000^{r}/ 60000^{nr}	Yes	B-Lys-thio-benzylester Pro-Phe-Arg-AMC casein	780	Disulfide-linked dimer via Cys at position 76
Granzyme B	CTLA 1/CCP 1	29 000	Yes/mar-ginal[d]	NF	700	
Granzyme C		27 000	No	NF	830	
Granzyme D		35 000–50 000	Yes	Succ-Ala-Phe-Lys-AMC	300	Highly glycosylated
Granzyme E		35 000–45 000	Marginal	NF	500	
Granzyme F		35 000–40 000	No	NF	750	
Granzyme G	CTLA 1/CCP 1	33 000	Marginal	NF	620	
Granzyme H	CTLA 1/CCP 1	31 000	Marginal	NF		

AMC, aminomethylcoumarin; *NF*, no substrate found at present
[a] Based on the predicted amino acid sequences of the esterases encoded by the H factor clone (GERSHENFELD and WEISSMANN 1986) and clone CTLA 1/CCP 1 (BRUNET et al. 1986; LOBE et al. 1986b)
[b] As determined by SDS-PAGE. Only the apparent mass of granzyme A changed when electrophoresis was carried out under reducing (r) versus nonreducing (nr) conditions
[c] Only the best-cleaved substrates are indicated
[d] Depending on isolation conditions of the granule proteins

reducing conditions. The disulfide bond formation is due to cys-76, a surface-located cysteine which is not found in other serine proteases (e.g., trypsin, chymotrypsin), as will be discussed later. Granzyme C is the protease that elutes last from the Mono S column at 820 mM NaCl; it has the lowest apparent molecular mass (27 K) of all granzymes, suggesting the absence of carbohydrate moieties.

3 Substrates and Inhibitors of Granzymes

The identification of proteins as serine proteases is often achieved by using the serine esterase affinity label [³H] diisopropylfluorophosphate ([³H] DFP). After the cleavage of the ester bond of [³H] DFP, a covalent [³H] DFP-esterase complex is formed which is subsequently detectable by fluorography. Using this approach, purified granzymes A and D are strongly labeled (Table 1) (MASSON and TSCHOPP 1987). Much weaker labeling is normally observed with granzymes B, E, G, and H. Granzymes C and F completely fail to associate with

Table 2. Relative amidase (esterase) activity of granzyme A

Substrate	Relative fluorescence units	Relative activity (%)
H-Pro-Phe-Arg-AMC	177.0	100
BOC-Val-Pro-Arg-AMC	59.4	34
BOC-Leu-Gly-Arg-AMC	8.8	5
Succ-Ala-Phe-Lys-AMC	18.1	10
BOC-Val-Leu-Lys-AMC	8.3	5
Succ-Gly-Pro-Leu-Gly-Pro-AMC	0.8	0
Succ-Ala-Ala-Ala-AMC	0.4	0
Succ-Ala-Ala-Pro-Val-AMC	4.1	2
H-Cys-Bzl-AMC	0.6	0
Absorbance$_{405}$		
N-α-Benzyloxycarbonyl-Lys-thiobenzylester (BLT)	0.86	100
Succ-Ala-Ala-Pro-Phe-thiobenzylester (SPT)	0.07	8
Absorbance$_{366}$		
Azocasein Granzyme A	0.26	4
Trypsin	0.907	100

AMC, aminomethylcoumarin. *BOC*, Butoxycarbonyl. *Bzl*, Benzoyl

the radioactive affinity label (MASSON and TSCHOPP 1987). Labeling of granzyme B with [³H] DFP is variable: whereas granzyme B is strongly labeled in whole lysates of B6.1 cells, of PC 60-induced cells (MASSON et al. 1986a), and of CTL lines tested by others (YOUNG et al. 1986f; TAKAYAMA and SITKOWSKY 1987a), it is only slightly labeled after purification (MASSON and TSCHOPP 1987). The reasons for this difference are unknown.

A panel of synthetic peptides has been tested as substrates for the granzymes. In agreement with the extent of the observed [³H] DFP labeling, substrates have only been found for granzymes A and D (MASSON and TSCHOPP 1987). The esterolytic activity of granzyme D, however, is very low relative to granzyme A, chymotrypsin, or trypsin. The best substrate found for granzyme D is Succ-Ala-Phe-Lys (Table 1). In contrast, granzyme A cleaves several synthetic substrates efficiently. Granzyme A shows trypsin-like activity in that it cleaves best after Arg or Lys (Table 2). The best synthetic substrates found are Pro-Phe-Arg-7-amino-4-methyl-coumarin or Pro-Phe-Arg-nitroanilide (SIMON et al. 1986, 1987; MASSON et al. 1986b) and BLT. Granzyme A also cleaves proteinaceous substrates such as casein (Table 2) or fibrin (YOUNG et al. 1986f). The pH optimum of granzyme A for the cleavage of the various substrates is around 8.0 (MASSON et al. 1986; SIMON et al. 1986).

The effect of several protease inhibitors on the esterolytic activity of granzyme A is shown in Table 3. Inhibitors of serine proteases like PMSF, aprotinin, leupeptin, DFP, and benzamidine are potent inhibitors (MASSON et al. 1986b; YOUNG et al. 1986f; SIMON et al. 1986). However, TLCK and TPCK, excellent inhibitors for trypsin and chymotrypsin, respectively, have no effect. The activity is also not dependent on the presence of metal ions.

Table 3. Inhibitors of granzyme A activity[a]

Enzyme inhibitor	Final concentration	Activity (% of control)
Control with DMSO		100
DFP	0.1 mM	0
PMSF	1 mM	3
	5 mM	1
Benzamidine	5 mM	0
SBTI	2 mg/ml	10
Aprotinin	0.1 mg/ml	2
Leupeptin	0.1 mg/ml	21
TPCK	1 mM	100
TLCK	1 mM	97
EDTA	1 mM	99
CaCl$_2$	1 mM	59
MgCl$_2$	0.01 mM	78
1,10-Phenanthroline	1 mM	93
Dithiothreitol	1 mM	41

DMSO, dimethyl sulfoxide; DFP, diisopropyl fluorophosphate; *PMSF*, phenylmethylsulphonyl fluoride; *SBTI*, soybean trypsin inhibitor; *EDTA*, ethylenediamine tetraacetic acid. *TPCK*, Tosyl-phenylalanyl-chloromethyl ketone; *TLCK*, Tosyl-lysyl-chloromethyl ketone
[a] Data taken from MASSON et al. (1986b), SIMON et al. (1986), and YOUNG et al. (1986f)

4 cDNA Cloning and Structural Features of Granzymes

The identification and structural analysis of the serine esterases found in cloned T-cell lines and induced peripheral blood mononuclear cells were greatly facilitated by the application of recombinant DNA techniques. The first clones shown to encode serine esterases of cytolytic T cells were isolated by subtraction screening techniques and with the use of cDNA subtraction libraries (BRUNET et al. 1986; LOBE et al. 1986a, b; GERSHENFELD and WEISSMANN 1986). Hybridization was performed with an excess of nonradioactive mRNA from a noncytolytic T-cell tumor line or a B-lymphoma line to compete with the single-stranded radioactive cDNA probe prepared from total poly (A$^+$) RNA of the cytolytic T-cell line. Other investigators have screened CTL-specific subtraction libraries with the two pools of reversely transcribed mRNA from noncytolytic and cytolytic T-cell clones in order to identify mRNA transcripts that were exclusively expressed in CTL lines. Those cDNA clones hybridizing with the radioactive cDNA pool from the cytolytic T cells, but not with that from noncytolytic T cells, were selected and analyzed by nucleotide sequencing. By this technique, three novel serine proteases expressed in T lymphocytes, the human lymphocyte protease and two murine proteases, granzyme A (H-factor, CTLA-3) (GERSHENFELD and WEISSMANN 1986; BRUNET et al. 1986) and granzyme B (CTLA-1, CCPI) (BRUNET et al. 1986; LOBE et al. 1986a), have been cloned.

The approach described above has certain limitations. Rare mRNA transcripts are difficult to detect, and an unknown number of expressed genes are related to the activation rather than to the effector functions of cytolytic T cells. An alternative approach for the cloning of T-cell effector molecules is based on the isolation of proteins associated with cytoplasmic granules, which are released upon target cell recognition. Partial amino acid sequences are determined for the purified proteins in order to design synthetic oligonucleotides for hybridization screening. Specific antibodies prepared against the purified granule proteins are another valuable tool used to screen cDNA expression libraries in lambda phage vectors or plasmid vectors.

The antibody screening approach utilized by our group resulted in cDNA clones coding for the granzymes (MASSON and TSCHOPP 1987). In addition to granzymes A and B, the remaining murine granzymes C, D, E, and F have been cloned and their complete covalent structure described. Since the antibodies used for expression cloning cross-reacted among the different granzymes, identification was achieved by comparing the cDNA-derived amino acid sequences for granzymes with the first 20 N-terminal residues, as determined by amino acid sequence analysis. All granzyme cDNA clones contain the polyadenylylation signal AATAAA in the 3' untranslated region. The translation initiation sites of the mRNA transcripts have been reported for most of the granzymes. Except for granzyme A (CTLA-3, H-factor), all predicted granzyme sequences start with a very hydrophobic stretch of 18 amino acid residues (Fig. 2), which represents a typical signal peptide (VON HEIJNE 1986), indicating that granzymes are translocated across the lipid membrane into the rough endoplasmatic reticulum. All granzymes, except granzyme B, are encoded by mRNA transcripts of about the same size, 1100 bp, as determined by Northern blot analysis (BRUNET et al. 1987; SCHMID and WEISSMANN 1987; JENNE, unpublished data). The nucleotide sequences of granzyme A and granzyme B do not hybridize with each other under stringent conditions (0.1 × SSC, 65° C), as judged from the results of genomic Southern blots. The full-length cDNA probe of granzyme B, however, hybridizes to two bands of 1600 and 1100 bp respectively, in Northern blots from certain cell lines, whereas an oligonucleotide specific for granzyme B only recognizes the 1600 bp transcript (JENNE et al., unpublished data). The granzyme B cDNA probe may therefore hybridize to the mRNA of other granzymes even under the highly stringent hybridization conditions used in the studies published (BRUNET et al. 1987).

The granzyme B (G, H) (CCP1) nucleotide sequence has the highest homology with the nucleotide sequence of human lymphocyte protease (HLP) (73% at the nucleotide level), which was found to be expressed in three human CTL clones and in one helper T-cell clone (SCHMID and WEISSMANN 1987). HLP is probably the human homologue of granzyme B since the granzyme B probe does not recognize other highly related genes in Southern blot experiments. Granzymes A and B appear to exist as single copy genes in the mouse genome, as judged from the number of genomic restriction fragments to which the respective full length cDNA probes hybridize (BRUNET et al. 1987).

The primary structure for granzymes A to F has been determined by cDNA sequencing as shown in Fig. 2. The cDNA-derived protein sequences are most

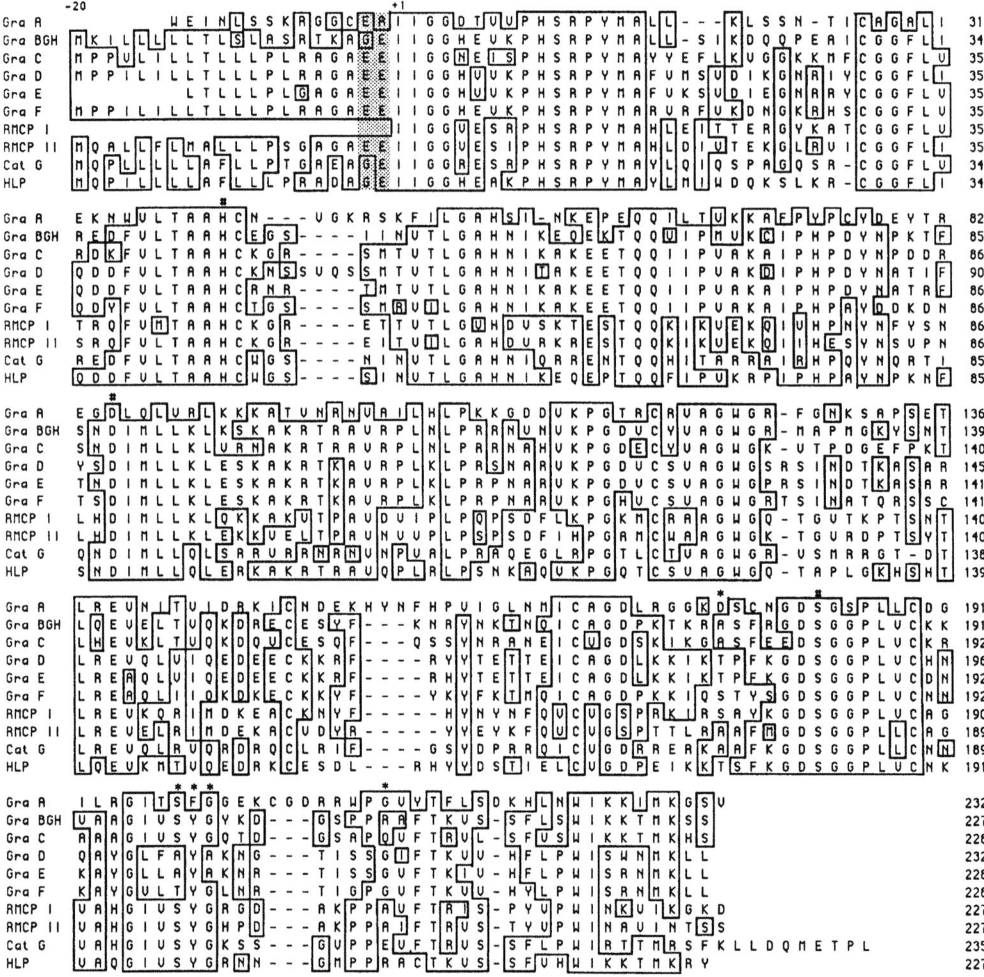

Fig. 2. The granzyme serine protease family. Amino acid sequences of all granzymes given in the single letter code have been aligned: *Gra A* (GERSHENFELD and WEISSMAN 1986), *Gra B* (BRUNET et al. 1986; LOBE et al. 1986b), *Gra C* (JENNE et al. 1988a), *Gra D* (JENNE et al. 1988b), *Gra E* (JENNE et al. 1988b), *Gra F* (JENNE et al. 1988b), human lymphocyte protease, *HLP* (SCHMID and WEISSMANN 1987), cathepsin G, *Cat G* (SALVESEN et al. 1987), rat mast cell protease I, *RMCP I* (TRONG et al. 1987), and rat mast cell protease II, *RMCP II* (BENFEY et al. 1987). *Dashes* indicate gaps introduced to maximize the sequence similarities among all granzymes. Residue numbering starts with the first amino acid residue of the mature granzymes as determined by amino acid sequencing (MASSON and TSCHOPP 1987) and is given at the end of each line. The two residues following the hydrophobic signal peptide form a short propeptide at the N-terminus of the granzymes and are emphasized by a *grey background*. Amino acid residues which are conserved in at least four of the ten proteins are surrounded by *boxes*. The residues histidine (*H*), aspartic acid (*D*), and serine (*S*), which form the catalytic site in serine proteases, are indicated by #. Residues lining the substrate binding pocket are found in positions −6, +15 to +17, and +25 relative to the active site serine in the aligned sequences (KRAUT 1977) and are marked by *stars*

closely related to rat mast cell protease II (RMCP) (Woodbury et al. 1978; Benfey et al. 1987) and cathepsin G (Salvesen et al. 1987) (at least 38% [granzyme A / RMCP II] positional identities), which are found in granules of differentiated mast cells and neutrophilic granulocytes, respectively, and show the typical features of novel serine protease in each case. Since the tertiary structure is highly conserved among proteins having overall sequence similarities of at least 20%, the protein folding of all granzymes can be predicted to resemble closely that of RMCP II. Gaps introduced at a few positions to maximize sequence similarities do not change the overall protein-folding pattern when these insertions or deletions are located on the surface of the homologous proteins within variable loops. Alignment of the amino acid sequences of granzymes to those of well-characterized members of the serine protease family (RMCP II, elastase, and trypsin) therefore permits the comparison of structural features of granzymes.

Two sequence features appear to be constitutive for this novel subfamily of serine proteases. First, the mature granzymes share a strictly conserved N-terminal sequence at residue positions $+1$ to $+4$ and positions $+9$ to $+16$ (Fig. 2) which is not found in other serine proteases. Second, they are synthesized as inactive precursor molecules with a very short acidic propeptide at the N-terminus consisting of either Gly-Glu or Glu-Glu. The pre-propeptide of granzyme A is not yet known and appears to be an exception, since its propeptide ends with Glu-Arg. Six cysteine residues are conserved among all family members and are linked together by disulfide bridges in a 1–2, 3–6, and 4–5 pattern analogous to the disulfide bonding pattern in RMCP II (Fig. 3). Granzyme A, however, contains a fourth cysteine bond at the C-terminus homologous to that of chymotrypsin, trypsin, and elastase (Woodbury and Neurath 1980). In addition, the free cysteine residue at position 76 gives rise to the formation of homodimers.

Glycosylation of granzymes shows enormous variation, ranging from granzyme C without carbohydrate moieties to granzyme D with a very large carbohydrate content of up to 50% of its molecular weight. Granzyme C does not appear to bear carbohydrate structures according to biochemical analysis and has no asparagine-linked glycosylation sites (Fig. 2). Granzyme D on the other hand shows the highest heterogeneity in molecular size, ranging from 35 K to 50 K, and contains five asparagine-linked glycosylation sites. Three glycosylation sites in equivalent positions are shared by granzymes D, E, and F. Granzymes D and E have the fourth glycosylation site in common. This site is in close proximity to the catalytic histidine. Glycosylation at this site has been reported in the case of cathepsin G (Salvesen et al. 1987), and thus the question arises whether glycosylation of this asparagine changes the enzymatic activity of granzymes D and E. The amounts of negatively charged carbohydrate moieties clearly influence the net charge of granzymes whose polypeptide chains are unusually basic. As discussed above, the isoforms of granzymes with the highest carbohydrate content elute first from the cation exchange column Mono S, and the lower molecular weight species (which have fewer carbohydrate moieties) thereafter. The degree of negatively charged carbohydrates attached to the polypeptide chain may also determine the stability and dissociation of com-

Gra A (H factor, CTLA-3)

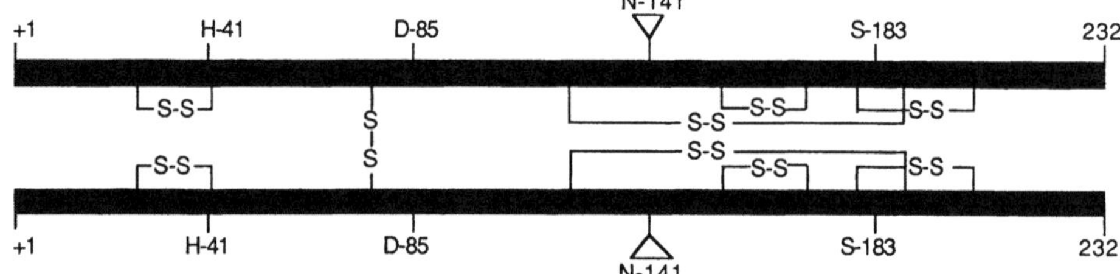

Gra B (CTLA-1, C11), C, D, E, F, HLP, Cat G, RMCP I/II

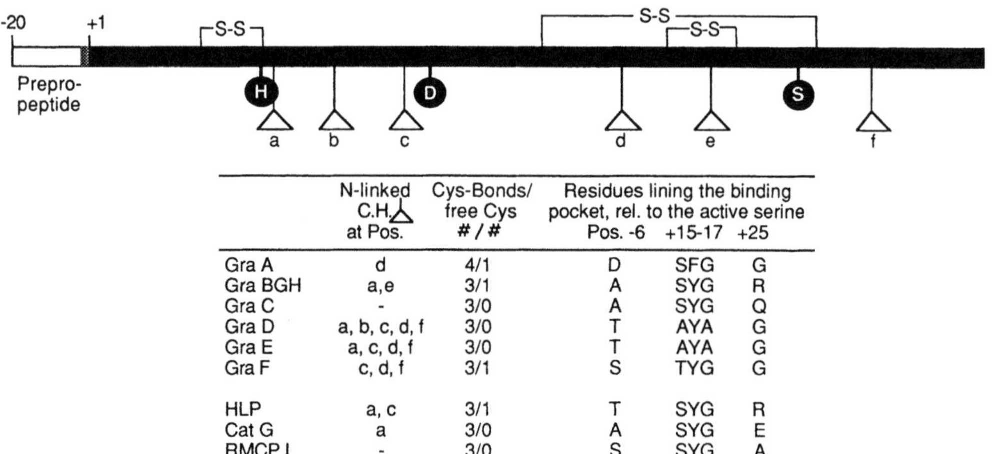

	N-linked C.H. at Pos.	Cys-Bonds/ free Cys # / #	Residues lining the binding pocket, rel. to the active serine		
			Pos. -6	+15-17	+25
Gra A	d	4/1	D	SFG	G
Gra BGH	a,e	3/1	A	SYG	R
Gra C	-	3/0	A	SYG	Q
Gra D	a, b, c, d, f	3/0	T	AYA	G
Gra E	a, c, d, f	3/0	T	AYA	G
Gra F	c, d, f	3/1	S	TYG	G
HLP	a, c	3/1	T	SYG	R
Cat G	a	3/0	A	SYG	E
RMCP I	-	3/0	S	SYG	A
RMCP II	-	3/0	A	SYG	A

Fig. 3. Structural features of granzymes. Except for *Gra A* (GERSHENFELD and WEISSMAN 1986; MASSON et al. 1986b) all granzymes, *Gra B* (BRUNET et al. 1986; LOBE et al. 1986b), *Gra C* (JENNE et al. 1988a), *Gra D* (JENNE et al. 1988b), *Gra E* (JENNE et al. 1988b), *Gra F* (JENNE et al. 1988b), human lymphocyte protease, *HLP* (SCHMID and WEISSMAN 1987), cathepsin G, *Cat G* (SALVESEN et al. 1987), rat mast cell protease I, *RCMP I* (TRONG et al. 1987), and rat mast cell protease II, *RMCP II* (BENFEY et al. 1987), show a highly homologous protein structure. The *solid black bar* represents the polypeptide chain of the mature enzymes; the *open bar*, the hydrophobic signal peptide; and the *grey segment*, the short propeptide. The numbering of the protein sequences starts with the first N-terminal residue (+1) of the mature enzymes as determined by amino acid sequencing (MASSON and TSCHOPP 1987). The location of the catalytic site residues, histidine (*H*), aspartic acid (*D*), and serine (*S*), the putative attachment sites for N-glycosylation (*triangles*), and the cysteine bond pattern are indicated *beneath* the bars. Granzyme A (*upper part*) is a homodimer with two active catalytic centers and one additional cysteine bond per polypeptide chain at the C-terminus. The protein structure of the remaining monomeric granzymes is shown schematically in the *lower part* of the drawing. For each of these granzymes, the *table at the bottom* lists the distribution of N-linked glycosylation sites, the number of cysteine bonds and free cysteine residues, and the amino acid residues (in single letter code) which are considered to determine the substrate specificity (KRAUT 1977)

plexes formed with the negatively charged chondroitin sulfate to which the basic granzymes are bound within the granules. Prolonged, continuous diffusion of granzymes into the interstitial fluid of tissues may depend on the variable degree of glycosylation.

Alignment of the amino acid sequences of granzymes also reveals similarities and some differences in functional properties regarding the substrate specificity. Although the key residues forming the catalytic center, histidine, aspartic acid, and serine, are strictly conserved and found at equivalent positions as in other serine proteases, some of the residues at positions -6, $+15$ to $+17$, and $+25$ relative to the active site serine, which are believed to determine the substrate specificity (KRAUT 1977), are different. By comparing these residues to those of well-characterized serine proteases like trypsin, chymotrypsin, and elastase, granzyme A was tentatively classified as trypsin-like, since it also contains an aspartic acid at the bottom of the substrate-binding pocket (position -6). In agreement with this prediction, granzyme A cleaves synthetic substrates best after an arginine, as has been already discussed. Granzymes B to F, however, differ considerably from the trypsin and chymotrypsin residue pattern and cannot be classified in such a simple way. Residue differences at the positions shown in Fig. 3 may therefore indicate novel, distinct substrate specificities. The respective residues are highly similar in granzymes D, E, and F, and in the case of granzymes D and E are even identical, suggesting a very similar or identical substrate specificity for these three granzymes. For granzymes B, C, E, and F, suitable synthetic substrates have not been identified. The intracellular sorting of murine granzymes and removal of the propeptide has not been studied. As for cathepsin G and RMCP II, it has been suggested that the propeptide is removed during or just before packaging into the cytoplasmic granules. Activation and storage of granzymes, therefore, may differ completely from that of trypsin and chymotrypsin, which are secreted from exocrine pancreas cells as zymogens.

5 Expression of Granzymes

Protein and mRNA expression has been studied so far only for the murine granzymes A, B, and C. Granzyme A was detected in various CTL lines, in nude mouse spleen (which contains many NK cells), in some helper T cell lines (CD4+, CD8−), and in NK-cell-derived tumor cell lines (GERSHENFELD and WEISSMAN 1986; BRUNET et al. 1987). Expression was not strictly correlated with the cytolytic activity of the cell types studied. Granzyme A mRNA was also identified in CD4+ and CD8+ subsets of mixed leukocyte cultures that had been cultured for 3–5 days in IL-2-supplemented growth medium (GARCIA-SANZ et al. 1987). Like granzyme A, granzymes B and C are expressed in cytotoxic T-cell clones and in NK-cell-containing nude mouse spleen cell populations (LOBE et al. 1986a). The published data, however, do not rule out the possibility that granzymes B and C can be synthesized as well by noncytolytic CD4+

helper cells under certain conditions, or transiently following specific stimulation. Sequences homologous to granzyme B have also been identified in murine mast cell populations and virus-transformed, murine mast cell lines (which seem to be cytotoxic) (BRUNET et al. 1987). Thus, the question arises whether mast cells express granzyme B transcripts in addition to the mast cell-specific serine proteases (BENFEY et al. 1987). The spectrum and identity of proteases found in murine mast cells, however, has not been studied, and cDNA sequences for the murine homologues of rat mast cell proteases I and II are not available.

Taken together, expression of granzyme B seems to be confined to T lymphocytes and mast cells exhibiting cytolytic activity, whereas granzyme A transcripts are also detected in noncytolytic cells. For the other granzymes, no or inadequate expression studies are available to draw conclusions from.

6   Function of Granzymes

The actual physiological functions of granzymes are not known. One or several of them may well be the proteases that are inactivated by the panel of protease inhibitors that abrogate CTL activity. All cytotoxic cells studied to date express granzymes. That granzyme A is also expressed in noncytotoxic cells is not an argument against a role in T-cell-mediated cytotoxicity. Upon conjugate formation with the target cell and exocytosis of the granule contents, granzymes and perforin may act synergistically on the target membrane: the former proteolyze membrane proteins, thereby facilitating insertion of perforin. That PMSF-treated granules or cells are as lytic as their nontreated counterparts (MASSON et al. 1986a) may suggest that granzyme A, the activity of which is abolished by PMSF, is not involved in the cytotoxic process.

Granzymes may also act after the actual delivery of the lethal protein. It is well-known that CTL, after conjugate formation and the delivery of toxic molecules, can detach and "recycle", i.e., continue on to lyse additional targets. The dissociation of effector and target cells may be mediated by granzymes, which would act on the various receptor and ligand molecules involved in CTL-target cell recognition and conjugate formation.

Granzyme A has been shown to cleave endothelial cell-derived extracellular matrix (SIMON et al. 1987). It may therefore allow stimulated T cells to invade and penetrate blood vessel walls, thereby facilitating their migration. Yet another role for granzyme A suggested by SIMON et al. (1986) is its involvement in B-cell growth. Earlier studies have shown that thrombin and trypsin can drive B cells to proliferation. This protease-induced B-cell growth may also be brought about by granzyme A.

Many other possible functions of granzymes may be envisaged. All of them can be tested now that the purification of substantial quantities of proteases has become possible. Study of the cDNA-derived primary structure may also clarify their three-dimensional structures based on the X-ray data collected for RMCP II (REYNOLDS et al. 1985). Hence, possible substrates and inhibitors may be predicted, allowing the identification of the physiological role of granzymes.

Acknowledgments. We thank Ms. Burnier, Mr. Freiwald, and Dr. R. Etges for help in preparing and editing the manuscript. D.E. Jenne is a recipient of a long-term EMBO fellowship.

References

Benfey PN, Yin FH, Leder P (1987) Cloning of the mast cell protease, RMCP II. J Biol Chem 262:5377–5384

Brunet J-F, Dosseto M, Denizot F, Mattei M-G, Clark WR, Haqqi TM, Ferrier P, Nabholz M, Schmitt-Verhulst A-M, Luciani M-F, Goldstein P (1986) The inducible cytotoxic T-lymphocyte-associated gene transcript CTLA-1 sequence and gene localization to mouse chromosome 14. Nature 322:268–271

Brunet J-F, Denizot F, Suzan M, Haas W, Mencia-Huerta J-M, Berke G, Luciani M-F, Goldstein P (1987) CTLA-1 and CTLA-3 serine esterase transcripts are detected mostly in cytotoxic T cells, but not only and not always. J Immunol 138:4102–4105

Chang TW, Eisen HM (1980) Effects of N-tosyl-l-lysyl-chloromethylketone on the activity of cytotoxic T lymphocytes. J Immunol 124:1028–1033

Garcia-Sanz JA, Plaetinck G, Velotti F, Masson D, Tschopp J, MacDonald HR, Nabholz M (1987) Perforin is present only in normal activated Lyt2$^+$ T lymphocytes and not in L3T4$^+$ cells, but the serine protease granzyme A (H-factor) is made by both subsets. EMBO J 6:933–938

Gershenfeld HK, Weissman IL (1986) Cloning of a cDNA for a T cell-specific serine protease from a cytotoxic T lymphocyte. Science 232:854–858

Hatcher VB, Oberman MS, Lazarus GS, Grayzel AI (1978) A cytotoxic proteinase isolated from human lymphocytes. J Immunol 120:665–670

Henkart PA, Millard PJ, Reynolds CW, Henkart MP (1984) Cytolytic activity of purified cytoplasmic granules from cytotoxic rat large granular lymphocyte tumors. J Exp Med 160:75–93

Hudig D, Haverty T, Fulcher C, Redelman D, Mendelsohn J (1981) Inhibition of human natural cytotoxicity by macromolecular antiproteases. J Immunol 126:1569–1574

Hudig D, Redelman D, Minning LL (1984) The requirement for proteinase activity for human lymphocyte-mediated natural cytotoxicity (NK): evidence that the proteinase is serine dependent and has aromatic amino acid specificity of cleavage. J Immunol 133:2647–2654

Jenne DE, Rey C, Masson D, Stanley KK, Herz J, Plaetinck G, Tschopp J (1988a) cDNA cloning of granzyme C, a granule-associated serine protease of cytolytic T lymphocytes. J Immunol 140:318–323

Jenne DE, Rey C, Haefliger J-A, Qiao B-Y, Groscurth P, Tschopp J (1988b) Identification and sequencing of cDNA clones encoding the granule-associated serine proteases granzyme D, E and F of cytolytic T-lymphocytes. Proc Natl Acad Sci USA 85:4814–4818

Kraut J (1977) Serine proteases: structure and mechanism of catalysis. Annu Rev Biochem 46:331–358

Lavie G, Leib Z, Servadio C (1985) The mechanism of human NK cell-mediated cytotoxicity. Mode of action of surface-associated proteases in the early stages of the lytic reaction. J Immunol 135:1470–1476

Lobe CG, Havele C, Bleackley RC (1986a) Cloning of two genes that are specifically expressed in activated cytotoxic T lymphocytes. Proc Natl Acad Sci USA 83:1448–1452

Lobe CG, Finlay BB, Paranchych W, Paetkau VH, Bleackley RC (1986b) Novel serine proteases encoded by two cytotoxic T lymphocyte-specific genes. Science 232:858–861

MacDermott RP, Schmidt RE, Caulfield JP, Hein A, Bartley GT, Ritz J, Schlossman SF, Austen KF, Stevens RL (1985) Proteoglycans in cell-mediated cytotoxicity. J Exp Med 162:1771–1787

Masson D, Tschopp J (1985) Isolation of a lytic, pore-forming protein (perforin) from cytolytic T-lymphocytes. J Biol Chem 260:9069–9072

Masson D, Tschopp J (1987) A family of serine esterases in lytic granules of cytolytic T-lymphocytes. Cell 49:679–685

Masson D, Corthésy P, Nabholz M, Tschopp J (1985) Appearance of cytolytic granules upon induction of cytolytic activity in CTL-hybrids. EMBO J 4:2533–2538

Masson D, Nabholz M, Estrade C, Tschopp J (1986a) Granules of cytolytic T-lymphocytes contain two serine esterases. EMBO J 5:1595–1600

Masson D, Zamai M, Tschopp J (1986b) Identification of granzyme A isolated from cytotoxic T-lymphocyte granules as one of the proteases encoded by CTL-specific genes. FEBS Lett 208:84–88

Millard PJ, Henkart MP, Reynolds CW, Henkart MP (1984) Purification and properties of cytoplasmic granules from cytotoxic rat LGL tumors. J Immunol 132:3197–3204

Nabholz M, MacDonald HR (1983) Cytolytic T lymphocytes. Annu Rev Immunol 1:273–306

Neurath H (1984) Evolution of proteolytic enzymes. Science 224:350–357

Pasternack MS, Eisen HN (1985) A novel serine esterase expressed by cytotoxic T lymphocytes. Nature 314:743–745

Pasternack MS, Verret CR, Liu MA, Eisen HN (1986) Serine esterase in cytolytic T lymphocytes. Nature 322:740–743

Podack ER (1985) The molecular mechanism of lymphocyte-mediated tumor cell lysis. Immunol Today 6:21–27

Podack ER (1986) Molecular mechanisms of cytolysis by complement and by cytolytic lymphocytes. J Cell Biochem 30:133–170

Podack ER, Königsberg PJ (1984) Cytolytic T cell granules. Isolation, structural, biochemical, and functional characterization. J Exp Med 160:695–710

Podack ER, Young JD-E, Cohn ZA (1985) Isolation and biochemical and functional characterization of perforin 1 from cytolytic T-cell granules. Proc Natl Acad Sci USA 82:8629–8633

Quan P-C, Ishizaka T, Bloom BR (1982) Studies on the mechanism of NK cell lysis. J Immunol 128:1786–1791

Redelman D, Hudig D (1980) The mechanism of cell-mediated cytotoxicity. I. Killing by murine cytotoxic T lymphocytes requires cell surface thiols and activated proteases. J Immunol 124:870–878

Reynolds RA, Remington SJ, Weaver LH, Fisher RG, Anderson WF, Ammon HL, Matthews BW (1985) Structure of a serine protease from rat mast cells determined from twinned crystals by isomorphous and molecular replacement. Acta Crystallogr B41:139–147

Salvesen G, Farley D, Shuman J, Przybyla A, Reilly C, Travis J (1987) Molecular cloning of human cathepsin G: structural similarity to mast cell and cytotoxic T lymphocyte proteinases. Biochemistry 26:2289–2293

Schmid J, Weissmann C (1987) Induction of mRNA for a serine protease and a β-thromboglobulin-like protein in mitogen-stimulated human leukocytes. J Immunol 139:250–256

Schmidt RE, MacDermott RP, Bartley G, Bertovich M, Amato DA, Austen KF, Schlossman SF, Stevens RL, Ritz J (1985) Specific release of proteoglycans from human natural killer cells during target lysis. Nature 318:289–291

Simon MM, Hoschützky H, Fruth U, Simon H-G, Kramer MD (1986) Purification and characterization of a T cell specific serine proteinase (TSP-1) from cloned cytolytic T lymphocytes. EMBO J 5:3267–3274

Simon MM, Simon HG, Fruth U, Epplen J, Müller-Hermelink HK, Kramer MD (1987) Cloned cytolytic T-effector cells and their malignant variants produce an extracellular matrix degrading trypsin-like serine proteinase. Immunology 60:219–230

Takayama H, Sitkovsky MV (1987) Antigen receptor-regulated exocytosis in cytotoxic T lymphocytes. J Exp Med 166:725–743

Takayama H, Trenn G, Humphrey W Jr, Bluestone JA, Henkart PA, Sitkovsky MV (1987) Antigen receptor-triggered secretion of a trypsin-type esterase from cytotoxic T lymphocytes. J Immunol 138:566–569

Trong HL, Parmelee DC, Walsh KA, Neurath H, Woodbury RG (1987) Amino acid sequence of rat mast cell protease I (chymase). Biochemistry 26:6988–6994

Tschopp J, Masson D, Stanley KK (1986) Structural/functional similarity between proteins involved in complement- and cytotoxic T-lymphocyte-mediated cytolysis. Nature 322:831–834

von Heijne G (1986) A new method for predicting signal sequence cleavage sites. Nucleic Acids Res 14:4683–4690

Woodbury RG, Neurath H (1980) Structure, specificity and localization of the serine preoteases of connective tissue. FEBS Lett 114:189–196

Woodbury RG, Katunuma N, Kobayashi K, Titani K, Neurath H (1978) Covalent structure of a group-specific protease from rat small intestine. Biochemistry 17:811–819

Young JD-E, Leong LG, Liu C-C, Damiano A, Cohn ZA (1986a) Extracellular release of lymphocyte cytolytic pore-forming protein (perforin) after ionophore stimulation. Proc Natl Acad Sci USA 83:5668–5672

Young JD-E, Hengartner H, Podack ER, Cohn ZA (1986b) Purification and characterization of a cytolytic pore-forming protein from granules of cloned lymphocytes with natural killer activity. Cell 44:849–859

Young JD-E, Podack ER, Cohn Z (1986c) Properties of a purified pore-forming protein (perforin 1) isolated from H-2-restricted cytotoxic T cell granules. J Exp Med 164:144–155

Young JD-E, Cohn ZA, Podack ER (1986d) The ninth component of complement and the pore-forming protein (perforin 1) from cytotoxic T cells: structural, immunological, and functional similarities. Science 233:184–190

Young JD-E, Liu C-C, Leong LG, Cohn ZA (1986e) The pore-forming protein (perforin) of cytolytic T lymphocytes is immunologically related to the components of membrane attack complex of complement through cysteine-rich domains. J Exp Med 164:2077–2082

Young JD-E, Leong LG, Liu C-C, Damiano A, Wall DA, Cohn ZA (1986f) Isolation and characterization of a serine esterase from cytolytic T cell granules. Cell 47:183–194

The Molecular Mechanism of Complement C9 Insertion and Polymerisation in Biological Membranes

K.K. STANLEY

1   Introduction   49

2   The Molecular Structure of C9   50

3   Events During C9 Insertion into the Bilayer   54
3.1   Formation of the C5b-8 Complex   54
3.2   Binding of C9 to C5b-8   56
3.3   Unfolding of C9 and Its Interaction with the Lipid Bilayer   58
3.4   Oligomerisation of C9 in the Membrane Attack Complex   59

4   Conclusions   61

References   62

1 Introduction

Rapid lysis of target cells by complement requires the presence of all five terminal complement components C5b, C6, C7, C8 and C9. Although early studies using aged sheep erythrocytes as a target cell suggested a minor role for C9 in this process (STOLFI 1968; HADDING and MÜLLER-EBERHARD 1969), the prevailing view now is that the formation of stable cytolytic complexes in fresh erythrocytes or bacteria absolutely requires the presence of C9. There is still, however, considerable debate about the molecular structure of the lytic complex and the actual cause of cell death. Morphological (HUMPHREY and DOURMASHKIN 1969; BHAKDI and TRANUM-JENSEN 1978) and biochemical (BHAKDI and TRANUM-JENSEN 1984) studies have shown that hollow cylindrical pore structures (membrane attack complexes, or MACs) containing a large amount of C9 relative to the other terminal complement components form on the surface of target cells. Since C9 can be induced to polymerise in vitro to form cylindrical structures with similar dimensions (TSCHOPP et al. 1982a), a natural conclusion is that complement lysis is caused by the ability of C9 to insert and polymerise within the bilayer to form hollow pore complexes. An alternative to the pore model postulates that C9 causes lysis by a detergent-like disruption of the lipid bilayer (ESSER et al. 1979). The morphologically observed lesions on this model are regarded as non-cytolytic byproducts of C9 insertion into the membrane (DANKERT and ESSER 1985). This model is most attractive as an explanation of the effects of complement on enveloped viruses which are not susceptible

European Molecular Biology Laboratory, Meyerhofstrasse 1, D-6900 Heidelberg, Federal Republic of Germany

Current Topics in Microbiology and Immunology, Vol. 140
© Springer-Verlag Berlin · Heidelberg 1988

to osmotic lysis. Neither mechanism provides a particularly satisfactory explanation for lysis of gram-negative bacteria, however, since morphologically distinguishable complexes have only been observed in the outer membrane, while disruption of the inner membrane has been shown to be the important step in lysis (WRIGHT and LEVINE 1981). An indirect effect of complement-activated phospholipases (TAYLOR and KROLL 1984) or membrane-depolarising effects of C9 fragments (DANKERT and ESSER 1986) are possible explanations for this remote action of C9. It is possible that all of these mechanisms of cytolysis are used by C9 to differing extents in the lysis of different target cells.

Common to each of these lytic mechanisms is the important first step of C9 insertion into the bilayer. This is absolutely dependent in biological membranes on the presence of C5b-8 as a receptor for C9 binding, and occurs concomitantly with a major conformational change in the C9 molecule (TSCHOPP et al. 1982a). A second important property of C9 (irrespective of its functional significance) is its ability to polymerise into partial or complete tubular structures which form the basis of the observed morphological lesion. In this review I shall try and identify molecular properties of the terminal complement components, in particular C9, which may be associated with these two steps in MAC formation.

2 The Molecular Structure of C9

Human C9 is a glycoprotein of 538 amino acid residues with an apparent molecular weight on SDS gels of 71 000 daltons. Although the initial sequencing studies suggested only 537 amino acids (DISCIPIO et al. 1984; STANLEY et al. 1985), an additional valine at position 293 has been found on all cDNA and genomic clones except the first cDNA isolated (MARAZZITI et al. 1988). All numberings of amino acids in this review will therefore be with respect to this amended sequence (Fig. 1).

The gene for C9 is unusually long (>80 kb) and is situated on chromosome 5 of the human genome (K.K. STANLEY, unpublished data). It is expressed principally in liver and appears to be induced in some pathological conditions (RUMFELD et al. 1986; OLEESKY et al. 1986). The gene is composed of at least 11 exons (MARAZZITI et al. 1988) encoding a protein with five putative domains. The first two of these (domains 1 and 2 in Fig. 2) have been identified by sequence homology studies with other serum or plasma membrane proteins. At the amino terminus is a span of 77 amino acids containing 6 cysteine residues which is also found twice in C8α, C8β, and C7, and 3 times in each polypeptide chain of thrombospondin (HAEFLIGER et al. 1987; RAO et al. 1987; HOWARD et al. 1987; DISCIPIO et al. 1987; LAWLER and HYNES 1986). Using computer-predicted secondary structure algorithms, this segment is likely to fold into α- and β-structures interconnected by disulphide bonds (domain 1, Fig. 2). In contrast, the next region of the protein containing 6 cysteine residues in 40 amino acids is predicted to contain principally coil and turn regions between

```
  1 QYTTSYDPELTESSGSASHIDCRMSPWSEWSQCDPCLRQMFRSRSIEVFGQFNGKRCTDA
                              Domain 1
 61 VGDRRQCVPTEPCEDAEDDCGNDFQCSTGRCIKMRLRCNGDNDCGDFSDEDDCESEPRPP
                              Domain 2
121 CRDRVVEESELARTAGYGINILGMDPLSTPFDNEFYNGLCNRDRDGNTLTYYRRPWNVAS
                    Domain 3
181 LIYETKGEKNFRTEHYEEQIEAFKSIIQEKTSNFNAAISLKFTPTETNKAEQCCEETASS
                                                    Hinge
241 ISLHGKGSFRFSYSKNETYQLFLSYSSKKEKMFLHVKGEIHLGRFVMRNRDVVLTTTFVD
                              Domain 4
301 DIKALPTTYEKGEYFAFLETYGTHYSSSGSLGGLYELIYVLDKASMKRKGVELKDIKRCL

361 GYHLDVSLAFSEISVGAEFNKDDCVKRGEGRAVNITSENLIDDVVSLIRGGTRKYAFELK

421 EKLLRGTVIDVTDFVNWASSINDAPVLISQKLSPIYNLVPVKMKNAHLKKQNLERAIEDY
                              Domain 5
481 INEFSVRKCHTCQNGGTVILMDGKCLCACPFKFEGIACEISKQKISEGLPALEFPNEK
```

Fig. 1. The deduced amino acid sequence of complement component C9 showing the boundaries of the putative domains

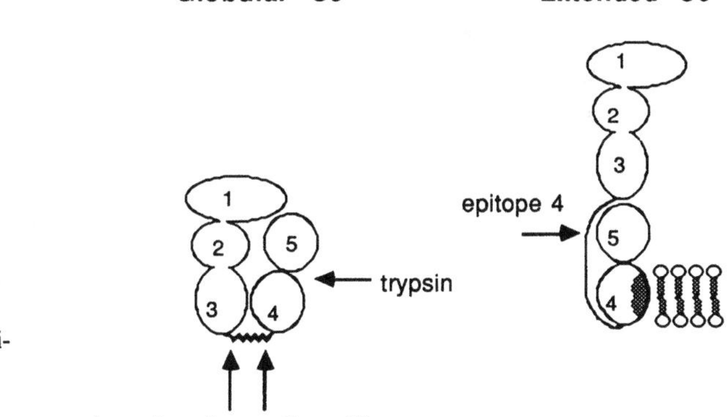

Fig. 2. A domain model of C9 in globular and extended conformations showing the proteolytic cleavage sites accessible only in globular C9 and the epitope (number 4, STANLEY and HERZ 1987) accessible only in extended C9

cysteine residues in common with structurally defined cysteine-rich domains in wheat germ agglutinin and erabutoxin (DRENTH et al. 1980; WRIGHT 1977; STANLEY et al. 1986). This sequence, called the class A cysteine-rich motif (domain 2, Fig. 2), is also found once in C7, C8α, and C8β; twice in factor I; seven times in the low density lipoprotein (LDL) receptor (SÜDHOF et al. 1985); and ten times in a putative apolipoprotein E receptor (HERZ et al. 1987). It is likely that this sequence folds into a small globular domain with the hydrophobic disulphide bonds buried at the centre and the connecting loops exposed at the surface as is found in other cysteine-rich domains (WRIGHT 1977). These sequences, which can be found in multiple copies, in general encode independently folding structural motifs of a protein and in some (SÜDHOF et al. 1985) but not all cases (MARAZZITI et al. 1988) are contained on discrete exons suggesting that they have been dispersed between different genes by exon shuffling. Near the C-terminus of C9 (residues 487–521) is a sequence showing a partial homology to the EGF precursor (class B) group of cysteine-rich sequences (DOOLITTLE 1985; STANLEY et al. 1986). It most clearly resembles the sequence found in urokinase, especially at the C-terminal end of the homology. At the present time there are insufficient data to describe this as a separate domain, especially as the 20 K fragment containing this sequence within it and corresponding to domain 5 in Fig. 2 is very stable to trypsin digestion.

Protease digestion experiments suggest two particularly labile sites (YAMAMOTO and MIGITA 1981; BIESECKER et al. 1982; Fig. 2) one occurring roughly in the centre of the molecule (characteristic of α-thrombin cleavage) and the other about 20 K from the C-terminus (characteristic of trypsin cleavage). These accessible cleavage sites fall between domains 3/4 and 4/5, respectively (Fig. 2). After a single cleavage by either α-thrombin or trypsin the molecule remains intact but separates into two fragments on non-reducing SDS gels, showing that non-covalent forces bind the domains together in globular C9. Nicking C9 in this way with α-thrombin leaves haemolytic activity intact, but with trypsin the haemolytic activity can actually be potentiated 2.4-fold as a result of removing a lag phase (TSCHOPP et al. 1986a).

Studies using iodinated C9 showed that after extensive trypsin digestion of MACs an 18 K fragment of C9 was left in the membrane (HAMMER et al. 1977). More recently, membrane-restricted, photoactivatable probes have been used to identify the position of this domain as between the α-thrombin and trypsin cleavage sites and contained on two CNBr fragments (AMIGUET et al. 1985; SCHÄFER et al. 1987). Examination of the sequence of C9 in three different species suggests that this is a region of close homology surrounded by areas of divergence (STANLEY and HERZ 1987). These data together suggest a separate domain (number 4 in Fig. 2) containing the lipid-interacting areas of C9.

Thus C9 probably contains five regions with some measure of independent folding (Fig. 2), consistent with the beaded appearance of C9 in negative-stained electron micrographs, especially after detergent treatment (PODACK and TSCHOPP 1982a, b). It is possible that the first two regions are tightly apposed in one 'domain' since proteolytic cleavage does not easily occur between them. Together they might form the 'torus' seen in electron micrographs of poly-C9. Little is known about the 3rd and 5th putative domains, but since these are relatively stable to protease digestion it is likely that they fold in a globular rather than extended structure.

These data on the domain structure of C9 pertain to the globular plasma form of the molecule, which is accessible to proteases. After insertion into the

MAC a large conformational change occurs, as shown by the loss of sensitivity to chymotrypsin and trypsin (YAMAMOTO and MIGITA 1981; PODACK and TSCHOPP 1982a), the loss of some antibody epitopes (MOLLNES and TSCHOPP 1987) and the gain of other epitopes (BHAKDI et al. 1975; KOLB and MÜLLER-EBERHARD 1975; PODACK et al. 1982; FALK et al. 1983; MOLLNES et al. 1985) and an apparent doubling in the length of the C9 molecule (PODACK and TSCHOPP 1982b). Particularly intriguing about the conformational rearrangement within the C9 molecule is that electron micrographs show the MAC to interact at the tip of the cylindrical complex, presumably by aggregation of the exposed hydrophobic, membrane-inserting domain (TSCHOPP et al. 1982a). Indeed, negatively-stained and freeze-etched electron micrographs of MACs in lipid vesicles did not show the MAC traversing the whole thickness of the bilayer (BHAKDI and TRANUM-JENSEN 1978; TRANUM-JENSEN and BHAKDI 1983). This is in contrast to the biochemical data cited above which show that the region of the polypeptide chain physically in contact with the lipid bilayer is almost at the centre of the molecule (domain 4, Fig. 2). A possible way around this dilemma is the proposal (STANLEY and HERZ 1987) that one region of the C9 molecule unwinds during the transition from globular to extended C9 allowing an unusual rearrangement of the globular domains (Fig. 2). This model is supported by: (a) the low conservation of sequence in the 'hinge' region consistent with a simple 'unravelling' function (STANLEY and HERZ 1987); (b) the presence in this region of two proteolytic sites and one epitope characteristic of only one form of the molecule (globular or extended); (c) the relatively small change in circular dichroism between the two structures (TSCHOPP et al. 1982a), suggesting that the rearrangement is principally between globular domains; and (d) the accessibility of epitopes in domains 1 and 5 from the extracellular space (McAb C9-42 and McAb C9-47, MORGAN et al. 1984; STANLEY and HERZ 1987).

The cartoon in Fig. 2 combines most of the available molecular data describing the different forms of C9 but is not intended as a precise drawing of the molecule. One small conflict is the observation that antibodies raised against the C9b fragment bind close to the torus of the MAC in negative-stained images (DiSCIPIO and HUGLI 1985) suggesting a less globular structure. It would clearly be of interest to map the epitopes of these antibodies more precisely.

A large number of surface features of the C9 molecule have been mapped to short regions of the polypeptide chain. These include (a) the site of attachment of N-linked oligosaccharides (STANLEY et al. 1985); (b) the sites of cleavage by chymotrypsin, α-thrombin and trypsin (STANLEY et al. 1985); (c) seven epitopes found in polyclonal antisera raised against C9 (STANLEY and HERZ 1987); and (d) the positions of deletions found in the sequences of C9 in different species and introns in the human C9 gene (MARAZZITI et al. 1988). The last category of features are not necessarily surface features but are not usually found buried in a protein where changes in sequence could cause major conformational changes. Hopefully this detailed topography will enable functional surfaces of the molecule to be determined using antibody and peptide inhibition experiments, or by site-directed mutagenesis.

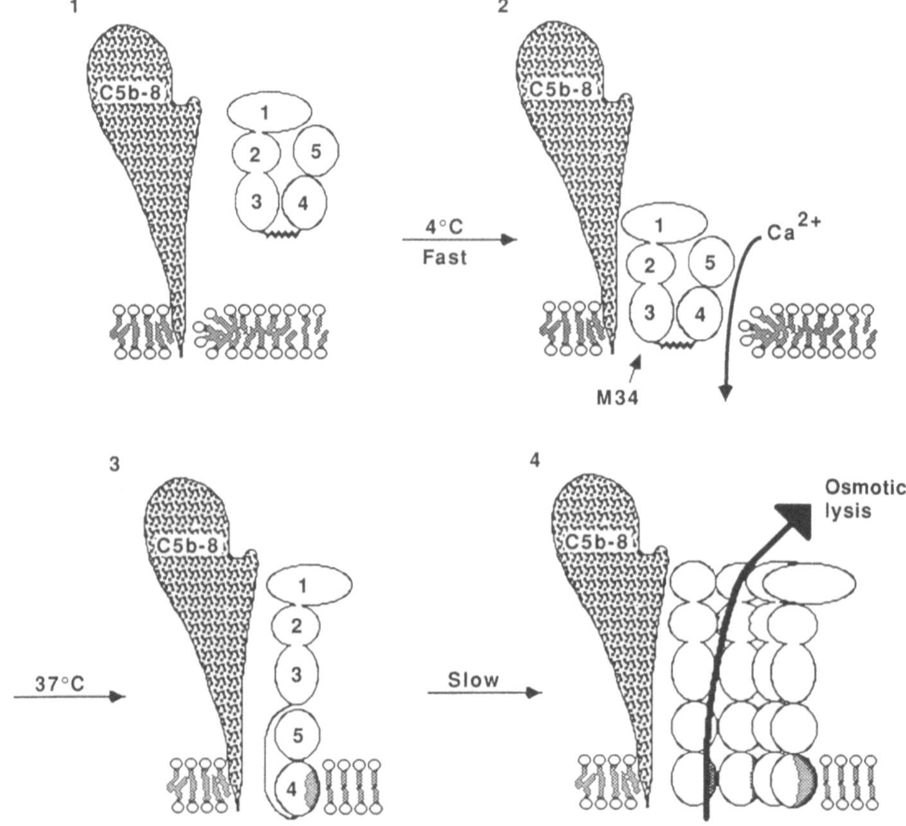

Fig. 3. A model for the insertion and polymerisation of C9

3   Events During C9 Insertion into the Bilayer

Several steps have been identified during C9 insertion into a target membrane. These are shown in cartoon form in Fig. 3.

3.1   Formation of the C5b-8 Complex

In order to understand the process of C9 binding to its receptor, C5b-8, it is necessary to understand the molecular nature of the individual components and how they interact in the assembled complex in the target membrane. Considerable progress has been made in the understanding of the individual molecules in the C5b-8 complex by the cloning and sequencing of all but C6. This has revealed that C7, C8α, and C8β are related to C9, having an overall homology starting at the N-terminus and running over the whole length of C9, but with one or more additional C-terminal domains (Fig. 4; HAEFLIGER et al. 1987;

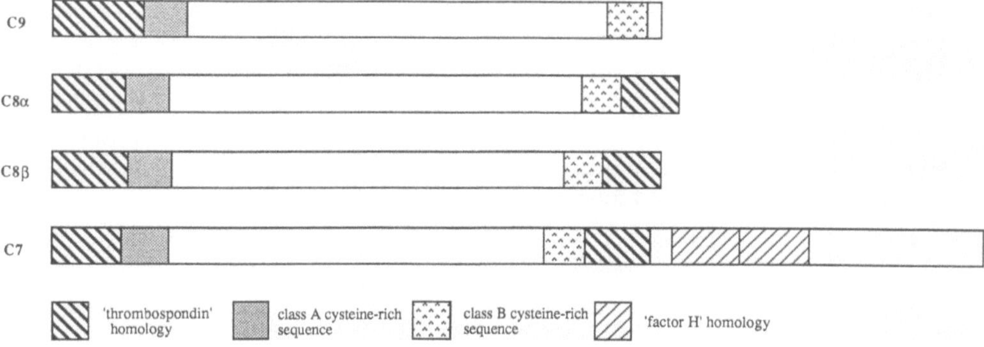

Fig. 4. Homologous regions in the terminal complement proteins

RAO et al. 1987; HOWARD et al. 1987; DISCIPIO et al. 1987). C8α and C8β both have a C-terminal extension of about 50 amino acids which is related to a sequence motif at the N-terminus of the proteins (domain 1) and a repeating sequence within thrombospondin (DISCIPIO et al. 1987; LAWLER and HYNES 1986). C7 also contains this sequence immediately following the C9 homologous region (Fig. 4) but in addition has a large, cysteine-rich, C-terminal extension containing two repeats of the motif found in C4-binding protein, factor H and the complement receptors CR1 and CR2 (SCHULZ et al. 1986). It is very likely that the C4-binding protein homology is involved in C7 interaction with C5b, and a similar sequence would be expected in the related protein C6.

C7, C8 and C9 are all globular serum proteins which change in conformation on interaction with the MAC (PODACK et al. 1979) and may be labelled at some point in MAC formation by membrane-restricted, photoactivatable probes (PODACK et al. 1981). It is likely that these similar properties are encoded by the major part of the sequence which is homologous. The ordered sequence of binding, on the other hand, may be determined by their additional C-terminal domains; in particular, that shared by C8α, C8β and C7 is found repeated three times in thrombospondin in a region which is responsible for binding the three chains of the molecule together (LAWLER and HYNES 1986), suggesting a possible interaction in this region which maintains the structure of the C5b-8 receptor. C9, which is similar to C8α and C8β except that it lacks this region, is able to polymerise in the MAC and form a stable pore. Insights into the structure-function relationships of this family of cytolytic proteins should also come from the sequence of perforin, a cytolytic protein expressed in natural and T killer lymphocytes. This protein shows antigenic (TSCHOPP et al. 1986b) and sequence (LOWREY et al. 1987) relationships to C9 but is different in that (a) it is packaged in secretory granules and released only after contact between effector and target cell, and (b) it appears to have no requirement for a receptor, specificity being conferred by the specificity of the effector:target cell interaction. These two properties are very likely to be linked, as the evolution of a cytolytic protein which is constitutively secreted would have to be accompanied by the development of a mechanism for controlling the cytolytic action. In this case it appears that gene duplication has occurred at least twice, and all the related gene products in the MAC are required for efficient lysis. C8 also has a subunit, C8γ, which is not homologous to C9. This is however related to the α_1-microglobulin family, one member of which has been shown to inhibit neutrophil chemotaxis (MENDEZ et al. 1986), suggesting a protective mechanism against amplification of the inflammatory response following complement attack on a host cell membrane (LUZIO and STANLEY 1988).

3.2 Binding of C9 to C5b-8

The nature of the molecular interaction during binding of C9 to the C5b-8 complex is not understood. From biochemical and kinetic studies it is known that the interaction is rapid at 4° C and occurs with the C9 in its globular conformation (SILVERSMITH and NELSESTUEN 1986 a, b). Direct binding studies between individual components have suggested that C8α can interact with C9 in buffers of physiological salt concentration (MONAHAN et al. 1983), although this is difficult to equate with the possible molecular interactions occurring in the membrane environment of the MAC between C5b-8 and C9. By using C5b-8 bound to filters, TSCHOPP and MASON (1987) were able to show an effect of suramine on C9 binding, implying an interaction between the LDL receptor homologies found in domain 2 of C7, C8α, C8β and C9, since suramine can dissociate apolipoprotein ligands from the LDL receptor (SCHNEIDER et al. 1982). The second domain in the terminal complement components contains regions resembling both the positively charged ligand and the negatively charged receptor (Fig. 5), thus allowing the possibility of lateral ligand-receptor-like interactions between adjacent molecules. If this hypothesis is correct, then the interaction cannot precisely mimic that of the LDL receptor with its ligand since C9 would then also bind to the LDL receptor itself (especially as C9 binds to the LDL receptor in a ligand blot) and thereby cause the lysis of all cells expressing the LDL receptor.

Although C5b-8 accelerates C9 polymerisation (TSCHOPP et al. 1985), kinetic studies in vitro do not support a decrease in the activation energy for polymerisation of C9 in the presence of C5b-8 which might be expected for a direct catalysis (SILVERSMITH and NELSESTUEN 1986a). Attempts to cross-link C9 to the C5b-8 have also failed (MONAHAN et al. 1983), despite the fact that C8 is essential for C9 binding to the MAC. An alternative hypothesis (STANLEY et al. 1986) is that C9 simply inserts into holes in the lipid bilayer created by C5b-8, which is known to disturb the lipid bilayer (McCLOSKY et al. 1986), or into dislocations present in bilayers of low surface pressure or small radius of curvature (ESSER et al. 1985; TSCHOPP et al. 1982a, b). In this context C9 might have a more general role in immune surveillance, inserting into and destroying cells unable to maintain an intact plasma membrane.

Irrespective of the initial means of binding, studies using a C9 monoclonal antibody called M34 or (McAb C9-34) have suggested that C9 bound at 4° C to C5b-8 exists in a globular state at a site deeply embedded in the membrane

A

```
Human LDL receptor
          4-44      DRCER-NEFQCQD--GKCISYKWVCDGSAECQDGSDESQETCLS
                    -+ -+   -       -     +      +    -   -  -  --   -
         45-85      VTC-KSGDFSCGGRVNRCIPQFWRCDGQVDCDNGSDEQG--CPP
                        +   -       + +        + -    -  -    --
         86-124     KTC-SQDEFRCHD--GKCISRQFVCDSDRDCLDGSDEAS--CPV
                    +       -- +  -    +    +      - -+-  -   --
        125-165     LTC-GPASFQCN--SSTCIPQLWACDNDPDCEDGSDEWPQRCRG

        174-212     SPC-SAFEFHCL--SGECIHSSWRCDGGPDCKDKSDEEN--CAV
                        -            -         + -    -  +-+  ---
        213-251     ATC-RPDEFQCSD--GNCIHGSRQCDREYDCKDMSDEVG--CVN
                        + --     -            +   -+-  - +-   --
        253-294     TLCEGPNKFKCH--SGECITLDKVCNMARDCRDWSDEPIKECGT
                     -   + +       -      -+      +- +-  --   +-


B
Human C9  78-115    DDC--GNGFQCS--TGRCIKMRLRCNGDNDCGDFSDEDD--CES
                    --                + + + +   - -  -  ----   -
Mouse C9            ENC--GNDFQCE--TGRCIKRRLLCNGDNDCGDYSDEND--CDD
                    -       -    -    + +++      - -  -  -- -   --
Trout C9            SEC-SSIEFTCE--SGACIKLRLSCNGDYDCEDGSDED---CEP
                    -       -    -    + +        - - --  ---    -

C
Human C9  415-425                    YAFELKEKLLR
                                      - +-+   +
Mouse C9                             QAILLKEKILR
                                      +-+   +
Trout C9                             AAVAMRTQITK
                                      +     +

D
Apo E     140-150                    HLRKLRKRLLR
                                     ++ +++   +
Apo B     3357-3367                  TTRLTRKRGLK
                                      +  +++   +
```

Fig. 5 A–D. Comparison of the charged regions of C9 with those of the LDL receptor and apolipoproteins: **A** apolipoprotein binding site of the LDL receptor, **B** positively and negatively charged regions in domain 2 of C9, **C** positively charged region in domain 5 of C9, and **D** positively charged, receptor-binding region of apolipoproteins E and B

(step 2 in Fig. 3). This antibody (a) binds to a DTT-sensitive, discontinuous epitope in the N-terminal half of C9 (STANLEY et al. 1985), (b) inhibits the Zn^{2+}-catalysed polymerisation of C9. MALDONADO and STANLEY unpublished material) and (c) prevents sucrose efflux from erythrocyte ghosts if it is added inside the ghosts but not if it is added externally (MORGAN et al. 1984). These data suggest that an N-terminal portion of C9 must be transiently exposed to the cytoplasmic space and that M34 prevents efflux by inhibiting unfolding and polymerisation of the C9. The lack of photoactivatable probe labelling (HU et al. 1981) and the trypsin sensitivity of C9 bound to C5b-8 at 0° C support the idea that C9 binds in its globular state without direct interaction with the bilayer. Such an insertion of globular C9 into the bilayer could also account for the rapid effects of C9 on calcium ion permeability (CAMPBELL and LUZIO 1981; CAMPBELL et al. 1981).

3.3 Unfolding of C9 and Its Interaction with the Lipid Bilayer

After binding to C5b-8 complexes on erythrocytes at 4° C, the C9 remains in the trypsin-sensitive state characteristic of globular C9. Only after warming up the cells does lysis occur. If trypsin is added after warming up the cells for a short time, no inhibition of haemolysis is observed (BOYLE et al. 1978), suggesting that the C9 either becomes inaccessible or changes conformation shortly after the temperature shift. Since it is known that polymerised C9 is very resistant to protease digestion it is tempting to conclude that the C9 molecule refolds at 37° C into a protease-resistant, extended conformation (step 3 in Fig. 3). Trypsin-insensitive C9 cannot be equated with the formation of poly-C9 tubules, however, since it is formed before any release of markers or haemolysis of the erythrocytes (BOYLE et al. 1978). A slow conformational change of C9 after binding is also supported by kinetic studies (SILVERSMITH and NELSESTUEN 1986a, b).

When C9 is compared with apolipoprotein E (apo E), the region of highest homology falls in the sequence of apo E that interacts with the LDL receptor (STANLEY and HERZ 1987). The corresponding part of C9 has a similar motif of positive charges and leucine residues (Fig. 5c, d). Thus C9 in the globular state may be stabilised by an intramolecular ligand-receptor-like interaction between domains 2 and 5 (STANLEY and HERZ 1987). An antibody raised against the apo E homologous region of C9 does not bind to C9 in its globular conformation (R.O. LAINE and A.F. ESSER, personal communication), showing that this region is most likely involved in an intramolecular contact. After unfolding it is proposed that the positively and negatively charged regions on the second domain of C9 might interact with those on C8α (or other extended C9 molecules) in order to stabilise the complex.

Unfolding of C9 must also expose or generate a membrane-interacting site since globular C9 shows no tendency to bind lipids or detergents as compared with C9 in C5b-9 complexes (PODACK et al. 1979; TSCHOPP et al. 1984), and is the principal component of the MAC labelled by membrane-restricted, photoactivatable probes (HU et al. 1981; PODACK et al. 1981; ISHIDA et al. 1982; STECKEL et al. 1983; AMIGUET et al. 1985); this suggests a direct interaction with the acyl chains of the lipid bilayer. Biochemical studies have narrowed down the area of intact C9 labelled by the membrane-restricted, photoactivatable probe TID to two short sequences, residues 245–272 and 273–346, defined by the α-thrombin cleavage site (residue 245) and two CNBr cleavage sites (residues 272 and 346; SCHÄFER et al. 1987), showing that the polypeptide chain must traverse the bilayer at least twice. Since 12 molecules of C9 can form a cylindrical complex enclosing a 10-nm channel, each C9 molecule must occupy about 2.9 nm of circumference. This again suggests that several transmembrane segments are involved. In the first TID-labelled fragment, residues 245–267 (corresponding to the 'hinge' region in Fig. 2) are poorly conserved between species. This leaves only the predicted helical region 268–289 for interaction with the bilayer (STANLEY et al. 1986; SCHÄFER et al. 1987). In the second TID-labelled fragment, residues 292–326 can be folded into an amphipathic helix, although only a part of this is predicted using preference parameters for soluble proteins. This amphipathic structure is conserved in the different species of C9 and in human C8α, C8β and C7. Also conserved is Pro–306 in the centre of the sequence, which could be accommodated in the centre of a membrane-spanning segment (RAO and ARGOS 1986) or initiate a turn separating two transmembrane segments. It is of interest that His–324 is also a conserved amino acid in all the terminal components, as a histidine is often found at the surface of the lipid bilayer (RAO and ARGOS 1986). Residues 309–326 are particularly well conserved in the C9 sequences from distant species indicative of an important structural or functional role (STANLEY and HERZ 1987). It has been suggested that this sequence would have the interesting property of only folding when buried in the bilayer, thus making C9 interaction with the bilayer effectively irreversible (STANLEY and HERZ 1987). The only other hydrophobic sequence in the TID-labelled fragment consists of residues 337–341 which would have to assume a β-sheet structure in order to span the bilayer. Surprisingly, the whole region labelled by TID is quite charged, and it is difficult to understand how C9 binds so tightly to the lipid bilayer. Whether two α-helices, or three helices and a segment of β-sheet are involved in the membrane-interacting domain of C9, only between 4 and 12 amino acids would be present on the cytoplasmic face of the membrane, accounting for the difficulty in observing this part of the protein under the electron microscope.

Energy for the unfolding of C9 is presumably required since C9 remains in its trypsin-sensitive, globular state at 4° C (BOYLE et al. 1978). Some stabilisation of the extended C9 could be derived from the interaction with C5b-8, other C9 molecules or the lipid bilayer, although the similar activation energy for assembly of C5b-9 in the fluid phase or lipid bilayer suggests that the bilayer interaction contributes little (SILVERSMITH and NELSESTUEN 1986b). The ability of trypsin cleavage to potentiate haemolysis and remove a lag phase during channel formation (TSCHOPP et al. 1986a) suggests that the rate-limiting step includes a reorganisation of the C9 molecule involving domains 4 and 5.

3.4 Oligomerisation of C9 in the Membrane Attack Complex

The C9 molecule has the ability in vitro to form dimers, polymers and aggregates, properties which are likely to reflect its interactions in the MAC. Freshly isolated C9 often contains some dimers, which may be present in a disulphide-linked form. Disulphide-linked C9 dimer has also been observed in MACs isolated from erythrocyte membranes and has been attributed to the presence of reduced glutathione in these cells (YAMAMOTO et al. 1982). It is not clear whether the C9 dimer is present in functional cytolytic complexes, and photoaffinity labelling studies using different probes have given contradictory results concerning the proximity of the C9 dimer to the lipid bilayer (STECKEL et al. 1983; AMIGUET et al. 1985). Although not a necessary step in MAC formation, the catalysis of intermolecular disulphide bonds by exogenously added glutathione shows that cysteine residues in adjacent C9 molecules are close together, especially when MACs are formed using an excess of C9 (presumably generating tubular complexes).

C9 will form linear aggregates in vitro after incubation at 37° C with 0.6 *M* guanidinium hydrochloride, 0.1 *M* octyl glucoside or 1.5% sodium deoxycholate (PODACK and TSCHOPP 1982b). Such aggregates could result from an intermolecular interaction between the apo E homology in domain 5 and the negatively charged LDL receptor homology in domain 2 (Fig. 5). Linear aggregates have also been observed when C9 is nicked with α-thrombin and then polymerised in vitro with $ZnCl_2$ or allowed to interact with C5b-8 on erythrocyte membranes (DANKERT and ESSER 1986).

With intact C9, incubation at 37° C in the presence of zinc ions causes the formation of tubular C9 polymers which resemble the ultrastructure of the MAC (TSCHOPP 1984b). Under optimal conditions all of the C9 will polymerise with concomitant loss of haemolytic activity, but the composition of the polymers is heterogeneous, about one-third being resistant to boiling in SDS (in buffers of physiological salt concentration), the remainder dissociating to monomers under these conditions (TSCHOPP 1984b). Even after purification of the SDS-resistant poly-C9 as a 27 *S* complex, molecular weight measurements and morphological studies indicate a range of complexes containing between 12 and 18 C9 molecules.

The number of C9 molecules required per C5b-9 complex to cause cell death in vivo is also variable. MACs isolated from erythrocyte target membranes lysed with whole serum usually contain an average of between 4 and 8 C9 molecules, depending on the species (KOLB and MÜLLER-EBERHARD 1974; BHAKDI and TRANUM-JENSEN 1984; SIMS 1983; STEWART et al. 1984), but an average of only one C9 has been reported to have a lytic effect (ROMMEL and MAYER 1973; BHAKDI and TRANUM-JENSEN 1986); with low ratios of target cells to serum or C9-supplemented serum a range of 6–12 C9 molecules per MAC can be found (BHAKDI and TRANUM-JENSEN 1984; TSCHOPP 1984a; SILVERSMITH and NELSESTUEN 1986b). In gram-negative bacteria an average of 3 or more C9 molecules are required for lysis in lysozyme-free serum irrespective of the number of complexes on the bacterial cell surface (BLOCH et al. 1987). Studies using the electron microscope suggest the presence of cylindrical MAC structures in target membranes although it is difficult to prove that death occurred as a result of individual structures. Some of these are closed, SDS-resistant cylinders very similar in morphology to poly-C9 but having an additional component in negative-stained images which is interpreted as the C5b-8 complex (TSCHOPP et al. 1982b). Boiling in SDS removes the C5b and C8β, but leaves C6, C7 and C8α associated with the C9 (PODACK 1984). Further evidence for a direct contribution of these components in the generation of a cylindrical pore comes from measurements of the permeability of erythrocyte membranes containing C5b-9 complexes with an average of only 1 C9 molecule (BHAKDI and TRANUM-JENSEN 1986). The effective pore size of 1-3 nm under these circumstances is difficult to reconcile with the single C9 molecule per complex unless the earlier components can also participate in forming the cylindrical wall of the MAC. This possibility is perhaps not surprising in view of their similar sequences.

The relevance of SDS-resistant poly-C9 has been the subject of controversy. The ability to achieve cytolysis in the apparent absence of morphologically recognisable MACs using low C9 concentration (BHAKDI and TRANUM-JENSEN

1986) or α-thrombin-nicked C9 (DANKERT and ESSER 1985) has shown that SDS-resistant poly-C9 is not an absolute requirement. On the other hand the activation energy for C9 polymerisation is similar to that for complement-mediated haemolysis of sheep red blood cells, consistent with the suggestion that polymerisation of C9 is the rate-limiting molecular event associated with formation of cytolytic lesions (SIMS and WIEDMER 1984). Furthermore, haemolysis can be blocked by small molecules, like suramin and heparin, which have a high positive or negative charge (TSCHOPP et al. 1986b; TSCHOPP and MASSON 1987). Since these compounds are able to compete for binding of apolipoproteins to the LDL receptor (SCHNEIDER et al. 1982; GOLDSTEIN et al. 1976), this suggests that ionic interactions of domain 2 are involved in haemolysis. Although suramin could be nonspecific in its effects, an inhibitory peptide derived from the natural inhibitor of C9 polymerisation, S-protein or vitronectin, has been shown to bind to the negatively charged C-terminus of the class A, cysteine-rich sequence motif, suggesting that this region is directly involved in the formation of the MAC (TSCHOPP et al. 1987). Thus polymerisation, if not the formation of SDS-resistant polymers, appears to be intimately associated with haemolysis. Terminal complexes which are not SDS-resistant contain fewer C9 molecules but appear to be similarly embedded in the target cell membrane (AMIGUET et al. 1985) and to cause lesions with similar morphology but intermediate size and permeability (TSCHOPP 1984a). A reasonable interpretation is that effective pore structures can be made by the C5b-8 complex in conjunction with between 1 and 18 C9 molecules. The size of pore and presumably the efficacy of killing are related to the relative amounts of target cells and serum and the nature of the target cells, including the possibility of protective mechanisms in nucleated cells (MORGAN et al. 1987).

4 Conclusions

The molecular structure of C9 affords some explanation of its ability to insert into membranes and polymerise. Since C9 has both LDL-receptor-like and apo-lipoprotein-E-like sequences in the class A, cysteine-rich sequence motif (domain 2), a working hypothesis is that intermolecular ligand-receptor interactions between adjacent C9 molecules could account for at least a part of the stability of polymerised C9. Thus, the overall process of C9 insertion and polymerisation may involve the exchange of an intramolecular ligand-receptor interaction between domains 2 and 5 in globular C9 for an intermolecular interaction between different parts of domain 2 in extended C9 molecules in the MAC. C9 insertion also provides a model for understanding the interaction of other proteins with lipid bilayers. While post-translational insertion of proteins is unlikely to utilise the same sequences as C9, the principle of establishing an electrostatic binding to a receptor, followed by a refolding of the protein in order to create hydro-phobic patches for lipid interaction, could be a commonly used mechanism for the transition of an aqueous globular protein into an integral membrane protein.

Acknowledgment. I would like to thank Paul Luzio for his comments on this manuscript and many helpful discussions.

References

Amiguet P, Brunner J, Tschopp J (1985) The membrane attack complex of complement: lipid insertion of tubular and nontubular polymerized C9. Biochemistry 24:7328–7334

Bhakdi S, Tranum-Jensen J (1978) Molecular nature of the complement lesion. Proc Natl Acad Sci USA 75:5655–5659

Bhakdi S, Tranum-Jensen J (1984) On the cause and nature of C9-related heterogeneity of terminal complement complexes generated on target erythrocytes through the action of whole serum. J Immunol 133:1453–1463

Bhakdi S, Tranum-Jensen J (1986) C5b-9 assembly: average binding of one C9 molecule to C5b-8 without poly-C9 formation generates a stable transmembrane pore. J Immunol 136:2999–3005

Bhakdi S, Bjerrum UJ, Rother U, Knüfermann H, Wallach DFH (1975) Immunochemical analyses of membrane bound complement. Detection of the terminal complex and its similarity to intrinsic erythrocyte membrane proteins. Biochim Biophys Acta 406:21–35

Biesecker G, Gerard C, Hugli TE (1982) An amphiphilic structure of the ninth component of human complement. J Biol Chem 257:2584–2590

Bloch EF, Schmetz MA, Foulds J, Hammer CH, Frank MM, Joiner K (1987) Multimeric C9 within C5b-9 is required for inner membrane damage to *E. coli* J5 during complement killing. J Immunol 138:842–848

Boyle MDP, Langone JJ, Borsos T (1978) Studies on the terminal stages of immune hemolysis. J Immunol 120:1721–1725

Campbell AK, Luzio JP (1981) Intracellular free calcium as a pathogen in cell damage initiated by the immune system. Experientia 37:1110–1112

Campbell AK, Daw RA, Hallett MB, Luzio JP (1981) Direct measurement of the increase in intracellular free calcium ion concentration in response to the action of complement. Biochem J 194:551–560

Dankert JR, Esser AF (1985) Proteolytic modification of human complement protein C9: loss of poly(c9) and circular lesion formation without impairment of function. Proc Natl Acad Sci USA 82:2128–2132

Dankert JR, Esser AF (1986) Complement-mediated killing of *Escherichia coli*: dissipation of membrane potential by a C9-derived peptide. Biochemistry 25:1094–1100

DiScipio RG, Hugli TE (1985) The architecture of complement component C9 and poly(C9). J Biol Chem 260:14802–14809

DiScipio RG, Gehring MR, Podack ER, Kan CC, Hugli TE, Fey GH (1984) Nucleotide sequence of cDNA and derived amino acid sequence of human complement component C9. Proc Natl Acad Sci USA 81:7298–7302

DiScipio RG, Chakravarti DN, Müller-Eberhardt HJ, Fey G (1988) The structure of human complement component C7 and the C5b-7 complex. J Biol Chem 263:549–560

Doolittle WF (1985) The genealogy of some recently evolved vertebrate proteins. Trends Biochem Sci 10:233–237

Drenth J, Low BW, Richardson JS, Wright C (1980) The toxin-agglutinin fold. J Biol Chem 255:2652–2655

Esser AF, Kolb WP, Podack ER, Müller-Eberhard HJ (1979) Molecular reorganization of lipid bilayers by complement: a possible mechanism for membranolysis. Proc Natl Acad Sci USA 76:1410–1414

Esser AF, Dankert JR, Hansen JP, Leung KP (1985) Membrane insertion of C9 requires non-ordered lipid bilayers. Complement 2:23

Falk RJ, Dalmasso AP, Kim Y, Tsai CH, Scheinman JI, Gewurz H, Michael AF (1983) Neoantigen of the polymerized ninth component of complement. J Clin Invest 72:560–573

Goldstein JL, Basu SK, Brunschede GY, Brown MS (1976) Release of low density lipoprotein from its cell surface receptor by sulphated glycosaminoglycans. Cell 7:85–95

Hadding U, Müller-Eberhard HJ (1969) The ninth component of human complement: isolation, description and mode of action. Immunology 16:719–735

Haefliger J-A, Tschopp J, Nardelli D, Wahli W, Kocher H-P, Tosi M, Stanley KK (1987) Complementary DNA cloning of complement component C8 beta and its sequence homology to C9. Biochemistry 26:3551–3556

Hammer CH, Shin ML, Abramovitz AS, Mayer MM (1977) On the mechanism of cell membrane damage by complement: evidence on insertion of polypeptide chains from C8 and C9 into the lipid bilayer of erythrocytes. J Immunol 119:1–8

Herz J, Hamann U, Stanley KK (1987) A liver mRNA with high homology to the LDL-receptor. J Cell Biol 105:236a

Howard ZOM, Rao AG, Sodetz JM (1987) Complementary DNA and derived amino acid sequence of the beta subunit of human complement protein C8: identification of a close structural and ancestral relationship to the alpha subunit and C9. Biochemistry 26:3565–3570

Hu V, Esser AF, Podack ER, Wisnieske BJ (1981) The membrane attack mechanism of complement: photolabeling reveals insertion of terminal proteins into target membranes. J Immunol 127:380–386

Humphrey JH, Dourmashkin RR (1969) The lesions in cell membranes caused by complement. Adv Immunol 11:75–115

Ishida B, Wisnieski J, Lavine CH, Esser AF (1982) Photolabeling of a hydrophobic domain of the ninth component of human complement. J Biol Chem 18:10551–10553

Kolb WP, Müller-Eberhard HJ (1974) Mode of action of C9: adsorption of multiple C9 molecules to cell-bound C8. J Immunol 113:479–488

Kolb WP, Müller-Eberhard HJ (1975) Neoantigens of the membrane attack complex of human complement. Proc Natl Acad Sci USA 72:1687–1689

Lawler J, Hynes RO (1986) The structure of human thrombospondin, an adhesive glycoprotein with multiple calcium-binding sites and homologies with several different proteins. J Cell Biol 103:1635–1648

Lowrey DM, Frupp F, Aebischer T, Grey P, Hengartner H, Podack ER (1987) Primary sequence homology between the effector molecules that mediate complement and T lymphocyte cytotoxicity. Ann Inst Pasteur Immunol 138:296–300

Luzio JP, Stanley KK (1988) Sequence homology of complement C8γ chain with α_1-microglobulin and its implication for C8 structure and function. Mol Immunol 25:513–516

Marazziti D, Eggertsen G, Fey GH, Stanley KK (1988) Relationships between the gene and protein structure in human complement component C9. Biochemistry (in press)

McClosky MA, Dankert JR, Esser AF (1986) Interaction of complement proteins with bilayer lipids visualised by freeze-etch electron microscopy. Fed Proc 45:1941

Mendez E, Fernandez-Luna JL, Grubb A, Leyva-Cobian F (1986) Human protein HC and its IgA complex are inhibitors of neutrophil chemotaxis. Proc Natl Acad Sci USA 83:1472–1475

Mollnes TE, Tschopp J (1987) A unique epitope exposed in native complement component C9 and hidden in the terminal SC5b-9 complex enables selective detection and quantification of non-activated C9. J Immunol Methods 100:215–221

Mollnes TE, Lea T, Harboe M, Tschopp J (1985) Monoclonal antibodies recognising a neoantigen of poly(C9) detect the human terminal complement complex in tissue and plasma. Scand J Immunol 22:183–195

Monahan JB, Stewart JL, Sodetz JM (1983) Studies of the association of the eighth and ninth components of human complement within the membrane-bound cytolytic complex. J Biol Chem 258:5056–5062

Morgan BP, Luzio JP, Campbell AK (1984) Inhibition of complement-induced [^{14}C] sucrose release by intracellular and extracellular monoclonal antibodies to C9: evidence that C9 is a transmembrane protein. Biochem Biophys Res Commun 118:616–622

Morgan BP, Dankert JR, Esser AF (1987) Recovery of human neutrophils from complement attack: removal of the membrane attack complex by endocytosis and exocytosis. J Immunol 138:246–253

Oleesky DA, Ratanachaiyavong S, Ludgate M, Morgan BP, Campbell AK, McGregor AM (1986) Complement component C9 in Grave's disease. Clin Endocrinol 25:623–632

Podack ER (1984) Molecular composition of the tubular structure of the membrane attack complex of complement. J Biol Chem 259:8641–8647

Podack ER, Tschopp J (1982a) Circular polymerisation of the ninth component of complement. J Biol Chem 257:15204–15212

Podack ER, Tschopp J (1982b) Polymerisation of the ninth component of complement (C9): formation of poly(C9) with a tubular ultrastructure resembling the membrane attack complex of complement. Proc Natl Acad Sci USA 79:574–578

Podack ER, Biesecker G, Müller-Eberhard HJ (1979) Membrane attack complex of complement: generation of high-affinity phospholipid binding sites by fusion of five hydrophilic plasma proteins. Proc Natl Acad Sci USA 76:897–901

Podack ER, Stoffel W, Esser AF, Müller-Eberhard HJ (1981) Membrane attack complex of complement: distribution of subunits between the hydrocarbon phase of target membranes and water. Proc Natl Acad Sci USA 78:4544–4548

Podack ER, Tschopp J, Müller-Eberhard HJ (1982) Molecular organization of C9 within the membrane attack complex of complement. J Exp Med 150:268–282

Rao AG, Howard ZOM, Ng SC, Whitehead AS, Colten HR, Sodetz JM (1987) Complementary DNA and derived amino acid sequence of the alpha subunit of human complement protein C8: evidence of a separate alpha messenger RNA. Biochemistry 26:3556–3564

Rao JKM, Argos P (1986) A conformational preference parameter to predict helices in integral membrane proteins. Biochim Biophys Acta 869:197–214

Rommel FA, Mayer MM (1973) Studies of guinea pig complement component C9: reaction kinetics and evidence that lysis of EAC1-8 results from a single membrane lesion caused by one molecule of C9. J Immunol 110:637–647

Rumfeld WR, Morgan BP, Campbell AK (1986) The ninth complement component in rheumatoid arthritis, Behçet's disease and other rheumatic diseases. Br J Rheumatol 25:266–270

Schäfer S, Amiguet P, Tschopp J (1987) Transmembrane channel formation by C9 and histones. Complement 4:220

Schneider WJ, Beisegel U, Goldstein JL, Brown MS (1982) Purification of the low density lipoprotein receptor, an acidic glycoprotein of 164,000 molecular weight. J Biol Chem 257:2664–2673

Schulz T, Schäble W, Stanley KK, Weiß E, Dierich MP (1986) Human complement factor H: isolation of cDNA and partial cDNA sequence of the 38 K tryptic fragment containing the binding site for C3b. Eur J Immunol 16:1351–1355

Silversmith RE, Nelsestuen GL (1986a) Fluid-phase assembly of the membrane attack complex of complement. Biochemistry 25:841–851

Silversmith RE, Nelsestuen GL (1986b) Assembly of the membrane attack complex of complement on small unilamellar phospholipid vesicles. Biochemistry 25:852–860

Sims PJ (1983) Complement pores in erythrocyte membranes. Analysis of C8/C9 binding required for functional membrane damage. Biochim Biophys Acta 732:541–552

Sims PJ, Wiedmer T (1984) Kinetics of polymerisation of a fluoresceinated derivative of complement protein C9 by the membrane-bound complex of complement protein C5b-8. Biochemistry 23:3260–3267

Stanley KK, Herz J (1987) Topological mapping of complement component C9 by recombinant DNA techniques suggests a novel mechanism for its insertion into target membranes. EMBO J 6:1951–1957

Stanley KK, Kocher HP, Luzio JP, Jackson P, Tschopp J (1985) The sequence and topology of human complement component C9. EMBO J 4:375–382

Stanley KK, Page M, Campbell AK, Luzio JP (1986) A mechanism for the insertion of complement component C9 into target membranes. Mol Immunol 23:451–458

Steckel EW, Welbaum BE, Sodetz JM (1983) Evidence of direct insertion of terminal complement proteins into cell membrane bilayers during cytolysis. J Biol Chem 258:4318–4324

Stewart JL, Monahan JB, Brickner A, Sodetz JM (1984) Measurement of the ratio of the eighth and ninth components of human complement on complement-lysed membranes. Biochemistry 23:4016–4022

Stolfi RL (1968) Immune lytic transformation: a state of irreversible damage generated as a result of the reaction of the eighth component in the guinea pig complement system. J Immunol 100:46–54

Südhof TC, Goldstein JL, Brown MS, Russell DW (1985) The LDL receptor gene: a mosaic of exons shared with different proteins. Science 228:815–822

Taylor PW, Kroll H-P (1984) Interaction of human complement proteins with serum-sensitive and serum-resistant strains of *E. coli.* Immunology 21:609–620

Tranum-Jensen J, Bhakdi S (1983) Freeze-fracture analysis of the membrane lesion of human complement. J Cell Biol 97:618–626

Tschopp J (1984a) Ultrastructure of the membrane attack complex of complement: heterogeneity of the complex caused by different degree of C9 polymerization. J Cell Biol 259:7857–7863

Tschopp J (1984b) Circular polymerization of the membranolytic ninth component of complement: dependence on metal ions. J Biol Chem 259:10569–10573

Tschopp J, Masson D (1987) Inhibition of the lytic activity of perforin and of late complement components by proteoglycans. Mol Immunol 24:907–913

Tschopp J, Müller-Eberhard HJ, Podack ER (1982a) Formation of transmembrane tubules by spontaneous polymerization of the hydrophilic complement protein C9. Nature 298:534–538

Tschopp J, Podack ER, Müller-Eberhard HJ (1982b) Ultrastructure of the membrane attack complex of complement: detection of the tetramolecular C9-polymerising complex C5b-8. Proc Natl Acad Sci USA 79:7474–7478

Tschopp J, Engel A, Podack ER (1984) Molecular weight of poly(C9). J Biol Chem 259:1922–1928

Tschopp J, Podack ER, Müller-Eberhard HJ (1985) The membrane attack complex of complement: C5b-8 complex as accelerator of C9 polymerization. J Immunol 134:495–499

Tschopp J, Amiguet P, Schäfer S (1986a) Increased hemolytic activity of the trypsin-cleaved ninth component of complement. Mol Immunol 23:57–62

Tschopp J, Masson D, Stanley KK (1986b) Structural/functional similarity between proteins involved in complement- and cytotoxic T-lymphocyte-mediated cytolysis. Nature 322:831–834

Tschopp J, Masson D, Peitsch M (1987) Molecular mechanisms of C9 polymerisation and its inhibition by S-protein. Complement 4:232

Wright CS (1977) The crystal structure of wheat germ agglutinin at 2.2 Å resolution. J Mol Biol 111:439–457

Wright SD, Levine RP (1981) How complement kills *E. coli*: location of the lethal lesion. J Immunol 127:1146–1151

Yamamoto K, Migita S (1981) Proteolysis of the monomeric and dimeric C5b-9 complexes of complement: alteration in the susceptibility to proteases of the C9 subunits associated with C5b-9 dimerization. J Immunol 127:423–426

Yamamoto K, Kawashima T, Migita S (1982) Glutathione-catalyzed disulfide-linking of C9 in the membrane attack complex of complement. J Biol Chem 257:8573–8576

The Isolation and Characterization of Two Cytotoxic T-Lymphocyte-Specific Serine Protease Genes

R.C. BLEACKLEY

1   Introduction   67
2   The Differential Method of Isolating Function-Related Genes   68
3   B10 and C11 are CTL Specific   69
4   B10 and C11 Expression Correlates with Cytolytic Activity   69
5   B10 and C11 Encode Serine Proteases   70
6   CCPI has an Unusual Substrate Specificity   70
7   CCPI is Contained Within Cytoplasmic Granules   72
8   Organization of the Genomic Versions of B10 and C11   72
9   CCPI and II are Structurally Similar   73
10   CCPI and II Intron Positions Define a New Serine Protease Subfamily   73
11   Intracellular Mechanism of CTL Activation   74
12   B10 and C11 are Induced Sequentially and Their Expression Controlled Transcriptionally   75
13   During CTL Activation the Chromatin Conformation Surrounding the B10 and C11 Genes Changes   75
14   Role of Granular Proteins in CTL-Mediated Lysis   76
15   Do Serine Proteases Play a Key Role in CTL-Mediated Lysis?   77
References   78

1   Introduction

The search for the molecules involved in cytotoxic T-cell-mediated lysis has been primarily conducted using two approaches. The first of these was immunological, in which potentially relevant molecules were identified by antibodies that interfered with lysis. Such studies suggested the involvement of a number of cell surface molecules in the process but largely their roles appeared to be at the level of target cell binding (MARTZ et al. 1983). Secondly, classical protein biochemistry was used to search for lytic components, resulting in the isolation of a number of potential candidates that are discussed elsewhere in this book. Although both lines of research have provided useful information, the identities and roles of many of the molecules involved remain a mystery.

In my laboratory a more general approach to study this problem has been employed. It is based on the concept that the ability of a cell to perform a specific function is controlled by the unique function-related proteins that it

Departments of Biochemistry and Immunology, University of Alberta, Edmonton, Alberta, T6G 2H7, Canada

Current Topics in Microbiology and Immunology, Vol. 140
© Springer-Verlag Berlin · Heidelberg 1988

expresses. It is therefore reasonable that activated, cytotoxic T cells would contain a set of proteins which are directly involved in their ability to lyse target cells to which they are bound. Furthermore, such cytotoxicity-related proteins would not be expressed in other cells including closely-related types. Consequently, a strategy was adopted to identify and isolate such cytotoxic thymus-dependent lymphocyte (CTL)-specific products. In this chapter, the characterization of two such CTL-specific genes and their protein products is presented.

2 The Differential Method of Isolating Function-Related Genes

In 1976 Hastie and Bishop postulated that each cell type expresses a number of high abundance mRNAs which are not present in other cells. These mRNAs would encode proteins necessary for that cell to perform its specialized function. Using recombinant DNA methods it is now possible to isolate such function-related mRNAs through the cloning of their corresponding cDNAs.

Based on Hastie and Bishop's seminal work, I reasoned that CTL must express a number of cytotoxicity-related proteins and their corresponding mRNAs. In order to identify such molecules a differential screening method was used to identify cDNAs which were only expressed in activated cytotoxic cells. This kind of approach has been used to isolate a number of cell type-specific genes including muscle (HASTINGS and EMERSON 1982) and brain (MILNER and SUTCLIFFE 1983), also a number of cell cycle-specific genes (HIRSCHHORN et al. 1984) and some growth factor-induced genes (COCHRAN et al. 1983). Recently, similar logic led to the development of a subtractive approach for the cloning of the T-cell antigen receptor genes (HEDRICK et al. 1984; YANAGI et al. 1984). Although differential screening was employed to isolate the genes described in this review, recent experience suggests that the subtractive method offers some significant advantages.

In these experiments I reasoned that the function-related mRNAs would not be expressed either in other T-cell subsets (as represented by helper T cells) or in unactivated thymocytes. Thus, a cDNA library generated from the cytotoxic T-cell line MTL2.8.2 (BLEACKLEY et al. 1982) was screened with probes synthesized from the mRNA of killer cells, helper cells, and thymocytes. Differential screening of 5000 cDNA clones yielded 36 CTL-specific clones after three rounds of analysis. We have concentrated primarily on two of these CTL-specific genes, B10 and C11. These were chosen on the basis of preliminary cross-hybridization analysis, which indicated that the two sequences were homologous (LOBE et al. 1986a). A similar approach involving the screening of a CTL cDNA library with radioactive CTL probe in the presence of cold, noncytotoxic T-cell RNA resulted in the isolation of another CTL-specific clone, AR10 (GERSHENFELD and WEISSMAN 1986). This belongs to the same family as C11 and B10 (see later). In addition, using the subtractive approach (T cells minus B cells) three CTL-specific genes (CTLA-1, 2, 3) were also isolated (BRUNET et al. 1986); however sequence analysis revealed that CTLA-1 and CTLA-3 correspond to AR10 and C11, respectively.

3 B 10 and C 11 are CTL Specific

The expression of B 10 and C 11 was analyzed in a variety of cell types including other T-cell subsets as well as lymphoid and nonlymphoid cells. To summarize, it has been possible to detect expression of B 10 and C11 in 13 of 13 CTL clones or cultures including the so-called T-helper-killer cells (TITE and JANEWAY 1984). It was not possible to detect either transcript in resting thymocytes, resting or activated B cells, macrophages, liver, brain, and fibroblasts. Interestingly, hybridomas derived from peritoneal exudate lymphocytes (PEL) (KAUFMANN and BERKE 1983), which have cytolytic properties, do not express either B 10 or C 11. It should be noted that these cells neither contain cytolytic granules nor express the perforin protein (BERKE 1987). This suggests that PEL have evolved a completely different mechanism for killing. Recently, it has been reported that freshly isolated PEL do express C11 (BRUNET et al. 1987); however, the positive hybridization signal observed in these studies could be due to contamination with other cell types. Significant levels of C11 expression were detected in one helper cell which lacks cytolytic activity. This may reflect a breakdown in the clear definition and differences between helpers and killers as cells have now been described which have both functions (TITE and JANEWAY 1984). Perhaps this cell line, D10, may be partly differentiated towards becoming a helper-killer, but still lacks some of the components which would make it a functional killer.

4 B10 and C11 Expression Correlates with Cytolytic Activity

Expression of B10 and C11 was monitored during the development of a cytotoxic response in vitro. Cells were stimulated on day 0, and on subsequent days cytotoxicity was measured in a chromium-release assay while mRNA levels were assayed by cytodot analysis (LOBE et al. 1986a). It was observed that the increase in cytolytic activity was closely paralleled by increased levels of C11 and B10 mRNA. Similarly, as cytotoxicity declined so did the steady state level of the mRNA. The peak of cytotoxicity was observed on day 4 whereas B10 and C11 expression peaked 12–24 h earlier. Although these results do not provide definitive proof that B10 and C11 are involved in cytotoxicity, this pattern of expression is exactly what one would expect for mRNAs which encode proteins involved in the cell's ability to kill.

In situ hybridization has now been used to demonstrate that C11 expression occurs in cells surrounding an allograft transplant which is being rejected (MUELLER et al. 1988). This result is important for two reasons. Firstly, it proves that C11 expression occurs in vivo and is not an artifact of in vitro manipulation of cell lines. Secondly, the increased number of cells surrounding the allogeneic versus the syngeneic tissue which express C11 transcripts suggests that increased C11 expression correlates with CTL activity in this in vivo situation.

5 B10 and C11 Encode Serine Proteases

B10 and C11 cDNAs were sequenced and open reading frames identified. The predicted protein sequences were screened against a data base, and a number of homologous proteins were found. All of the proteins which showed greater than 30% homology belonged to the family of serine proteases. In addition, for the C11 predicted protein the three active site residues His, Asp, Ser, which constitute the catalytic triad of active serine proteases, could be identified (LOBE et al. 1986b). It is therefore highly probable that the protein encoded by C11, named cytotoxic cell protein I (CCPI), is a serine protease. However, I believe that CCPI corresponds to granzyme B (MASSON and TSCHOPP 1987), and as far as is known no enzymatic activity has yet been demonstrated for this molecule.

In addition to the mature serine protease, the predicted CCPI sequence (shown as the upper line in Fig. 1) has an extra 20 amino acid residues at the N-terminus, suggesting that a portion of this sequence acts as a signal peptide to direct secretion or intracellular localization. Interestingly, in addition to this presumptive signal sequence, the gene sequence encodes two further amino acids than the mature protease. This suggests that CCPI is synthesized in an inactive or zymogen form by virtue of the presence of these extra residues. Thus, it would require the action of a dipeptidase in order to become enzymatically active and perform its function during CTL-mediated lysis. Intuitively one would expect this to occur upon binding to a target cell, but N-terminal sequence analysis of granzyme B reveals the absence of the "activation dipeptide" in the molecule after isolation from CTL granules (MASSON and TSCHOPP 1987). This would suggest that the dipeptide is removed during assembly of the granules (see below).

Although a full length B10 has not been isolated, the partial sequence predicts that it is also a serine protease. Indeed, the genomic version of B10 has now been isolated (see below), and sequence analysis reveals that it also contains the three catalytic triad residues which characterize other serine proteases (see lower line of Fig. 1). The protein encoded by B10 has been named CCPII. It is tempting to speculate that these proteases, together with Hanukah factor (GERSHENFELD and WEISSMAN 1986), are involved in a protease cascade mechanism operating in CTL-mediated lysis in a fashion similar to the complement cascade in humoral immunity (REID 1986). However, as stated above, the proteases may have already been activated prior to target cell binding; thus this cascade idea becomes less likely.

6 CCPI has an Unusual Substrate Specificity

The predicted CCPI sequence has been aligned with the sequences of chymotrypsin and trypsin (LOBE et al. 1986b). Although overall there is a high level of homology with CCPI, there are a number of important differences in key resi-

```
                                        I
CCPI   MetLysIleLeuLeuLeuLeuLeuThrLeuSerLeuAlaSerArgThrLysAlaGlyGluIleIleGlyGlyHisGluValLysProHisSerArgProTyrMetAlaLeuLeuSer   39
        *       *  *  *  *     *     *         *  *  *  *  *     *        *  *  *  *  *  *  *
CCPII  MetProProValLeuIleLeuLeuThrLeuLeuLeuProLeuArgAlaGlyAlaGlyGluGluIleIleGlyGlyAsnGluIleSerProHisSerArgProTyrMetAlaTyrTyrGluPhe   40

                                                                        II
CCPI   IleLysAspGlnGlnProGluAlaIleCysGlyGlyPheLeuIleArgGluAspPheValLeuThrAlaAlaHisCysGluGlySerIleIleAsnValThrLeuGlyAlaHisAsnIle   79
        *           *  *  *  *     *        *  *  *  *  *  *  *  *     *  *        *  *  *  *  *  *  *  *
CCPII  LeuLysValGlyGlyLysLysMetPheCysGlyGlyPheLeuValArgAspLysPheValLeuThrAlaAlaHisCysLysGlySerSerMetThrValThrLeuGlyAlaHisAsnIle   80
                                                                       ⇑
                                                                                   III
CCPI   LysGluGlnGluLysThrGlnGlnValIleProMetValLysCysIleProHisProAspTyrAsnProLysThrPheSerAsnAspIleMetLeuLeuLysLeuLysSerLysAlaLys   119
        *        *     *  *  *     *  *     *  *  *  *  *  *  *        *  *     *  *  *  *  *  *     *  *
CCPII  LysAlaLysGluGluThrGlnGlnIleIleProValAlaLysAlaIleProHisProAspTyrAsnProAspAspArgSerAsnAspIleMetLeuLeuLysLeuValArgAsnAlaLys   120
                                                                       ⇑
CCPI   ArgThrArgAlaValArgProLeuAsnLeuProArgArgAsnValAsnValLysProGlyAspValCysTyrValAlaGlyTrpGlyArgMetAlaProMetGlyLysTyrSerAsnThr   159
        *  *  *  *  *  *  *  *  *  *  *  *  *        *  *  *  *     *  *  *  *  *  *        *     *        *
CCPII  ArgThrArgAlaValArgProLeuAsnLeuProArgArgAsnAlaHisValLysProGlyAspGluCysTyrValAlaGlyTrpGlyLysValThrProAspGlyGluPheProLysThr   160

CCPI   LeuGlnGluValGluLeuThrValGlnLysAspArgGluCysGluSerTyrPheLysAsnArgTyrAsnLysThrAsnGlnIleCysAlaGlyAspProLysThrLysArgAlaSerPhe   199
        *  *  *     *  *  *  *  *  *        *  *  *        *  *     *     *  *     *  *     *  *     *  *     *  *  *
CCPII  LeuHisGluValLysLeuThrValGlnLysAspGlnValCysGluSerGlnPheGlnSerSerTyrAsnArgAlaAsnGluIleCysValGlyAspSerLysIleLysGlyAlaSerPhe   200

       IV
CCPI   ArgGlyAspSerGlyGlyProLeuValCysLysLysValAlaAlaGlyIleValSerTyrGlyTyrLysAspGlySerProProArgAlaPheThrLysValSerSerPheLeuSerTrp   239
        *  *  *  *  *  *  *  *  *  *        *  *  *  *  *  *  *  *     *  *  *     *  *     *  *     *  *     *  *     *  *
CCPII  GluGluAspSerGlyGlyProLeuValCysLysArgAlaAlaAlaGlyIleValSerTyrGlyGlnThrAspGlySerAlaProGlnValPheThrArgValLeuSerPheValSerTrp   240
                    ⇑
CCPI   IleLysLysThrMetLysSerSer   247
        *  *  *  *  *  *  *  *
CCPII  IleLysLysThrMetLysHisSer   248
```

Fig. 1. Homology between two CTL-specific serine proteases, CCPI (encoded by C11) and CCPII (encoded by B10). The *upper line* gives the sequence for CCPI predicted from the cDNA sequence of C11, while the *lower line* gives the sequence for CCPII based on the genomic DNA of B10. The three active site residues are marked by *arrows*; the positions of introns is shown above the CCPI sequence in *roman numerals*; identical residues are marked by an *asterisk*; and the N-terminal signal and activation peptides are *underlined*

dues which are thought to influence the structure of the binding pocket and hence substrate specificity. Strikingly, CCPI lacks the cysteines which in other serine proteases form a disulfide bond to stabilize the binding pocket. This suggests that CCPI will have a much more flexible binding pocket, and this in turn may lead to the recognition of quite a long peptide substrate sequence. The high level of homology with rat mouse cell protease type II (RMCPII) has allowed the use of computer-assisted molecular modelling to predict the three-dimensional structure of CCPI (MURPHY et al. 1988). This analysis confirms the initial prediction of an unusual binding specificity for CCPI and predicts that the substrate specificity of CCPI will be unique among serine proteases. Specifically the replacement of Ala-226 of RMCPII by an arginine in CCPI suggests that the latter's substrate would contain an acidic apartate or glutamate in the P1 position. Again it is worth noting that using classical protein purification methods a serine protease with an unusual substrate specificity has been identified in CTLs (MASSON et al. 1986).

7   CCPI is Contained Within Cytoplasmic Granules

Using a predictive algorithm, in combination with the molecular modelling studies, a number of potentially antigenic sequences were identified in CCPI (REDMOND et al. 1987). Synthetic peptides were prepared, coupled to a carrier, and used to prepare antibodies. Western blot analysis showed that peptide-specific antibodies detect a protein of molecular weight 26000 (29000 upon reduction) only in CTLs. These antibodies have now been used to localize the protein to cytoplasmic granules using immunocytological and subcellular fractionation methods (REDMOND et al. 1987). Upon interaction of a cytotoxic cell with its target, granules polarize to the contact surface between the two cells. It has therefore been hypothesized that, by fusing with the cytoplasmic membrane, the granules deliver cytolytic components to the target cell (KUPFER and DENNERT 1984; YANELLI et al. 1986).

8   Organization of the Genomic Versions of B10 and C11

Labelled B10 and C11 cDNAs were used to probe genomic libraries of mouse DNA in bacteriophage lambda. High stringency hybridization and washing conditions, previously defined by genomic Southern blot analysis, were used in order to decrease the possibility of "false" positives. Positive plaques were isolated, DNA prepared, and preliminary restriction maps determined (LOBE et al. 1988a). Two recombinant phage DNAs whose maps corresponded to B10 and C11 were identified. Subfragments of each of these were cloned into either pUC13 or M13 and subjected to dideoxy sequencing. By comparison with the cDNA sequence it was possible to determine the exon/intron organization of the C11 gene. In addition it was possible to predict the positions of the introns for B10 as it was already known, that B10 and C11 are very homologous. Each gene is interrupted by four introns. The homology between the two genes, which was noted in their 3' ends (LOBE et al. 1986a), is conserved throughout the coding portions of the whole genes. Exons 1–5 are 56%, 66%, 78%, 82% and 80% homologous, respectively. In the 3' regions of the C11 and B10 genes, where they seem to be more similar, the homology even extends to 85% in the fourth intron. Although the sequence, homology in the other introns is much lower, their positions within the coding regions are almost identical. Clearly the C11 and B10 genes are evolutionarily related to each other and most probably to the RMCPII gene also (BENFY et al. 1987). It will be of great interest to see how the other granular serine protease genes are organized.

9   CCPI and II Are Structurally Similar

In the absence of a full length cDNA encoding CCPII I have predicted the protein sequence by positioning the introns of the B10 gene in equivalent positions to those found with C11 (LOBE et al. 1988a) and RMCPII (BENFY et al. 1987). The predicted sequence of CCPII is shown, compared with CCPI, in Fig. 1. As originally presumed, CCPII appears to be an active serine protease as it contains the three characteristic active site amino acids. The two proteins are clearly very homologous, and all of the key residue changes cited for CCPI (LOBE et al. 1986b; MURPHY et al. 1988), which led to the conclusion of an unusual binding pocket, are also present in CCPII. These include the absence of a pair of cysteines thought to stabilize the binding pocket of other proteases, the presence of an alanine six residues upstream from the active site serine, and the replacement of Ser-Trp-Gly-216 in chymotrypsin with Ser-Tyr-Gly. However, it should be noted that the residue crucial for predicting an acidic substrate specificity (MURPHY et al. 1988) in CCPI (Arg-208) is replaced by a glutamine in CCPII. The primary translation products of both genes carry hydrophobic leader sequences, plus an extra two residues. For CCPI this putative "activation dipeptide" is Gly-Glu, while in CCPII it is Glu-Glu. By virtue of their strong cross-hybridization with B10, two more cDNAs have recently been isolated which appear to belong to this same family of serine proteases. A comparison of their predicted protein sequences with the N-terminal analysis of the granzymes (MASSON and TSCHOPP 1987) suggests that they encode granzymes E and F. The predicted activation-dipeptide is Glu-Glu in both cases. Thus CCPI appears to be distinct in its mode of activation, perhaps suggesting some unique role.

10   CCPI and II Intron Positions Define a New Serine Protease Subfamily

The exon/intron arrangements of many serine protease genes are known, and a number have recently been compared (ROGERS 1985). All, except the intron-less bacterial genes, encode the three catalytic triad residues on separate exons. In this regard CCPI and II are no exception; however, closer inspection reveals that the positions of the third intron in the CTL-specific genes were different from any others previously described. It has been observed that serine protease gene introns normally map to areas of variability as defined by differences – insertions or deletions) between eukaryotic and prokaryotic proteases, and in addition that these regions correspond to surface regions of the protein (CRAIK et al. 1983). The position of the third intron in both CCPI and II does not correspond to either a region of variability or to a surface loop (LOBE et al. 1988a). It was therefore concluded that CCPI and II and RMCPII share a common ancestor and belong to a new subfamily of serine protease genes.

The position of the first intron in the two CTL-specific protease genes is also worthy of note. In many known serine protease genes the activation peptide portion of the gene is interrupted by an intron (ROGERS 1985). Even though, in the case of CCPI and II, the zymogen portion is only two amino acids, this "rule" is still adhered to. Perhaps it is important to preserve some sequence plasticity, by intron sliding, in this functionally crucial region of the protein. Indeed the precise positioning of intron 1 in CCPII may provide a case in point (see below).

11 Intracellular Mechanism of CTL Activation

Most of the contributions to the section on CTL-mediated lysis focus on the actual lytic mechanism. Whether or not this lytic state is achieved is governed in large part by the genes which are induced in response to stimulation of the precursor CTL by antigen and lymphokines. Consequently, it is of paramount importance to understand the nature of the intracellular events which control gene expression in CTL.

Many studies on helper T cells have implicated a variety of cytoplasmic membrane events in the mechanism of activation. These include changes in ion fluxes, calcium levels, membrane potential, and phospholipid metabolism, which have recently been reviewed (GELFAND et al. 1987; ISAKOV et al. 1987). However, the results of these experiments have thus far failed to provide a link between antigenic stimulation and transcriptional activation. The alternative approach has been to focus directly on the nucleus through the isolation and characterization of genes activated in T helper cells by antigenic stimuli. This has led to the identification of a number of important regulatory DNA sequences and provided evidence for the involvement of regulatory proteins (FUJITA et al. 1986; DURAND et al. 1987). In addition, the effects of metabolic inhibitors on transcriptional induction of specific genes have provided important clues as to the mechanism of activation of T helper cell genes (SHAW et al. 1987; KRÖNKE et al. 1985) and have suggested how immunosuppressive drugs, such as cyclosporin A, may act (ELLIOT et al. 1984).

Very little is known about events leading to transcriptional activation in cytotoxic cells. Generally, the conclusions gleaned from the studies cited above are extrapolated to include activation of all T-lymphocyte subsets. However, recent evidence has indicated that, in CTL, induction of the IL2-receptor gene and the subsequent chain of events which occurs after IL2 is bound to its receptor do not appear to involve calcium fluxes (MILLS et al. 1985a, b) or phospholipids (KOZUMBO et al. 1987), thus suggesting that there may well be fundamental differences between activation of these two subsets of T lymphocytes. A research program has been initiated aimed at elucidating the elements which are involved in regulating the expression of CTL-specific genes. The results of these studies should provide vital clues to the link between the membrane events and their nuclear consequences occurring upon CTL activation.

12   B10 and C11 are Induced Sequentially and Their Expression Controlled Transcriptionally

In the initial analysis of the levels of B10 and C11 mRNA during the in vitro generation of a cytotoxic T-cell response, it was concluded on the basis of cytodot data that the two genes were coordinately induced (LOBE et al. 1986a). However, in this assay it is not possible to distinguish between two such closely related genes. When a similar experiment was conducted using Northern blots to monitor the level of the two mRNAs, a slightly different conclusion was reached as in this assay C11 ($\sim$1500 nucleotides) and B10 ($\sim$1000 nucleotides) mRNAs could be distinguished. C11 mRNA was detectable on day 2, its level peaked on day 3, and it was almost absent on day 4. B10 mRNA was undetectable on day 2, also reached its maximum on day 3, but was still very much in evidence on day 4. Thus it is now thought that C11 and B10 are sequentially, rather than coordinately, induced (LOBE et al. 1988b).

Most of the analyses of C11 and B10 expression have focussed on measurements of steady state levels of mRNA. However, this is not always a reflection of transcriptional activity as changes in mRNA stability can, in a number of cases (SHAW and KAMEN 1986), influence the steady state levels. Changes in the transcriptional activity of the C11 gene were therefore assayed in an in vitro, transcriptional, run-on assay. The increase in steady state level of C11 mRNA was found to correspond with the transcriptional activation of the C11 gene (LOBE et al. 1988b). It was therefore concluded that C11 gene expression, and also likely that of the B10 gene, is controlled at the level of gene activation.

13   During CTL Activation the Chromatin Conformation Surrounding the B10 and C11 Genes Changes

Chromatin in the region of genes which are being, or have the potential to be, expressed is relatively decondensed (WEISBROD 1982). This altered conformation renders the gene in question accessible to transcription factors and thus is a first step towards gene activation. The loosening of chromatin can be detected using low levels of DNAse, which preferentially degrades this accessible DNA. The DNase sensitivity of the B10 and C11 genes was examined in CTL lines and compared with that of cells which do not express B10 and C11 transcripts.

Nuclei were isolated from a number of cytolytic and noncytolytic T-cell lines and digested with increasing levels of DNase. The DNA was then purified from these nuclei, cut with the restriction enzyme *Bam*HI, fractionated on an agarose gel, transferred to nitrocellulose, and probed with a variety of radioactively labelled cDNA fragments. The decline in the intensity of the hybridizing band, as the concentration of DNase is increased, is a reflection of the sensitivity. Scanning densitometry was used to quantitate the results obtained using probes for two regions of the C11 gene, the B10 gene, and the β-globin gene (not expressed in CTL) on a CTL clone and on unactivated thymocytes. In killer cell lines the 5'-ends of the C11 and B10 genes were found to be more sensitive to nuclease digestion than the 3'-ends of C11 or the β-globin gene, whereas in thymocytes all four probes revealed an equal level of sensitivity. The difference in DNAse sensitivity between the 5'- and 3'-ends of the C11 gene in the cytotoxic line is interesting and is perhaps indicative of the presence of important regulatory sequences in the 5'-flanking region of the C11 gene. The contrasting results for C11 and B10, compared with β-globin, between thymocytes and CTL clones is further proof that expression of these two protease genes is controlled transcriptionally.

Within DNase-sensitive regions hypersensitive sites occur which are thought to correspond to regions close to the binding sites of regulatory proteins. DNase hypersensitivity studies revealed two such sites each for B10 and C11 in killer cell clones. One of these sites occurs in both genes very close to where it is believed transcription initiates, as revealed by primer extension analysis. The other two are located ~400 and ~1000 base pairs upstream for C11 and B10, respectively. Perhaps these regions are involved in either the tissue- or activation-specific regulation of these two genes. In the latter case they would represent the ultimate target for the secondary messages emanating from antigen- and/or IL2-binding to their respective receptors on the surface of the precursor CTL.

14   Role of Granular Proteins in CTL-Mediated Lysis

A number of lines of evidence suggest that the cytoplasmic granules of CTL play a direct role in target cell lysis. Upon binding of CTL to targets, the Golgi apparatus and also granules polarize towards the point of contact (KUPFER and DENNERT 1984). The granules appear to fuse with the cytoplasmic membrane of the killer cell and could therefore release their contents in a very high concentration close to the target cell. One problem with this model is that the granular proteins could also damage the CTL which released them. However, the internal membrane of the granules must be impermeable to the lytic effector molecules or else all CTL would be destroyed by their own granular components. By the mechanism of exocytosis the internal granular surface becomes a part of the outer membrane of the effector CTL in the region of the interaction with the target cell. Therefore, in this area the CTL is impermeable to its granular components and thus resistant to killing.

One of the granular components, perforin (PODACK and KONIGSBERG 1984) or cytolysin (HENKART et al. 1984), has been shown to be lytic in its own right. However, perforin-induced lysis is not accompanied by chromosomal DNA fragmentation within the target cell. Thus, it is thought that perforin/cytolysin-induced lysis is not physiologically relevant to true CTL-mediated lysis. Another granular component could pass through the transmembrane channel created by polyperforin to act on endogenous molecules within the target cell to induce lysis (RUSSELL 1983). The identity of this effector molecule still remains uncertain, but a serine protease with an unusual substrate specificity would be an appealling candidate for such an activator of a preprogrammed death signal when it entered the target cell.

15 Do Serine Proteases Play a Key Role in CTL-Mediated Lysis?

Early experiments suggested that serine proteases may play an important role in CTL-mediated lysis (REDELMAN and HUDIG 1980; CHANG and EISEN 1980). More recently, an increase in serine protease activity has been noted upon activation of CTL (PASTERNACK and EISEN 1985; KRAMER et al. 1986; YOUNG et al. 1986).

These experiments indicate that CCPI is expressed uniquely in CTL. In addition, expression of C11 correlates with the development of cytotoxic activity, and CCPI appears to be localized within granules of activated cytotoxic cells. These results clearly suggest that CCPI is a key player in the cytolytic mechanism, but still its role remains unclear. Serine proteases could play a role in the degranulation process or facilitate polyperforin insertion into the target cell membrane. The analogy with the complement cascade would suggest that CCPI is involved in the activation of perforin so that it can become inserted into the target cell membrane. Alternatively, it may be involved in the detachment of the CTL from its target. It could even be the molecule which finds its way into the target cell and activates the suicide signal. Clearly, we are at present unable to define the precise role of CCPI in cell-mediated cytotoxicity; however, a number of recent results suggest that proteases do indeed play a role in killing, notably from serine protease inhibitors, which have been shown to inhibit granule-mediated lysis (SIMON et al. 1987).

Further experiments using, for example, antisense RNA technology should provide the answers to the role played by each of the granular components in the mechanism of CTL-mediated lysis. However, this may still be a considerable way from a complete understanding of its molecular basis. There seems to be increasing evidence for alternative forms of killing in the absence of detectable levels of granules or degranulation (OSTERGAARD et al. 1987; TRENN et al.

1987; BERKE 1987). Such results have now prompted me to return to the CTL libraries in search of other potential components of the cytolytic machine.

Acknowledgments. This work was supported by the National Cancer Institute of Canada. The author would like to express his sincere thanks to the many individuals who have contributed to the research effort in his laboratory, notably Corrinne Lobe who was responsible not only for initiating this research program but also for much of the data presented. In addition valuable contributions have been made by POPI HAVELE, NANCY EHRMAN, BRENDA DUGGAN, CHRIS UPTON, MICHAEL MEIER, JENNIFER SHAW, CHANTAL FREGEAU, MARC LETELLIER, MARK REDMOND, MICHAEL MURPHY, BRETT FINLAY, MIKE JAMES, and VERN PAETKAU. Finally, I am extremely grateful to Beverly Bellamy for her patience and understanding in the preparation of this manuscript. R. CHRIS BLEACKLEY is an Alberta Heritage Foundation for Medical Research Scholar.

References

Benfy PN, Yin FH, Leder P (1987) Cloning of mast cell protease, RMCP II. J Biol Chem 262:5377–5384

Berke G (1987) An appraisal of some current thoughts on cytolytic T-lymphocyte killing mechanisms. Ann Inst Pasteur Immunol 138:304–308

Bleackley RC, Havele C, Paetkau V (1982) Cellular and molecular properties of an antigen-specific cytotoxic T lymphocyte line. J Immunol 128:758–767

Brunet JF, Dosseto M, Denizot F, Mattei MG, Clark WR, Haqqi TM, Ferrier P, Nabholz M, Schmitt-Verhulst, AM, Luciani MF, Golstein P (1986) The inducible cytotoxic T-lymphocyte-associated gene transcript CTLA-1 sequence and gene localization to chromosome 14. Nature 322:268–271

Brunet JF, Denizot F, Suzan M, Haas W, Mencia-Huerta JM, Berke G, Luciani MF, Golstein P (1987) CTLA-1 and CTLA-3 serine esterase transcripts are detected most readily in cytotoxic T cells, but not only and not always. J Immunol 138:4102–4105

Chang TW, Eisen H (1980) Effects of *N*-tosyl-L-lysyl-chloromethylketone on the activity of cytotoxic T lymphocytes. J Immunol 124:1028–1033

Cochran BH, Reffell AC, Stiles CD (1983) Molecular cloning of gene sequences regulated by platelet-derived growth factor. Cell 33:939–947

Craik CS, Rutter WJ, Fletterick R (1983) Splice junctions: association with variations in protein structure. Science 220:1125–1129

Durand BD, Bush MR, Morgan JG, Weiss A, Crabtree GR (1987) A 275 basepair fragment at the 5′ end of the interleukin-2 gene enhances expression from a heterologous promoter in response to signals from the T-cell antigen receptor. J Exp Med 165:395–407

Elliott JF, Lin Y, Mizel SB, Bleackley RC, Harnish DG, Paetkau V (1984) Induction of IL2 mRNA inhibited by cyclosporin A. Science 21:1439–1441

Fujita T, Shibuya H, Ohashi T, Yamanishi K, Taniguichi T (1986) Regulation of human interleukin-2 gene: functional DNA sequences in the 5′ flanking region for the gene expression in activated T lymphocytes. Cell 46:401–407

Gelfand EW, Mills GB, Cheung RK, Lee JWW, Grinstein S (1987) Transmembrane ion fluxes during activation of human T lymphocytes: role of Ca^{2+}, Na^+/H^+ exchange and phospholipid turnover. Immunol Rev 95:59–87

Gershenfeld HK, Weissman IL (1986) Cloning of a cDNA for a T cell-specific serine protease from a cytotoxic T lymphocyte. Science 232:854–858

Hastie ND, Bishop JO (1976) The expression of three abundance classes of messenger RNA in mouse tissue. Cell 9:761–774

Hastings KEM, Emerson CP (1982) cDNA clone analysis of six co-regulated mRNAs encoding skeletal muscle contractile proteins. Proc Natl Acad Sci USA 79:1553–1557

Hedrick SM, Nielson EA, Kaveler J, Cohen DI, Davis MM (1984) Sequence relationships between putative T-cell receptor polypeptides and immunoglobulins. Nature 308:153–158

Henkart PA, Millard PJ, Reynolds CW, Henkart MP (1984) Cytotoxic activity of purified cytoplasmic granules from cytotoxic rat large granular lymphocyte tumors. J Exp Med 160:75–93

Hirschorn RR, Aller P, Yuan ZA, Gibson CW, Baserga R (1984) Cell-cycle-specific cDNAs from mammalian cells comperature sensitive for growth. Proc Natl Acad Sci USA 81:6004

Isakov N, Mally MI, Scholz W, Altman A (1987) T lymphocyte activation: the role of protein kinase C and bifurcating inositol phospholipid signal transduction pathway. Immunol Rev 95:89–111

Kaufman Y, Berke G (1983) Monoclonal cytotoxic T lymphocyte hybridoma capable of specific killing activity, antigenic responsiveness and inducible interleukin secretion. J Immunol 131:50–56

Kozumbo WJ, Harris DT, Gromkowski S, Cerottini JC, Cerutti P (1987) Molecular mechanisms involved in T cell activation. J Immunol 138:606–612

Kramer MD, Binninger L, Schirrmacher V, Moll H, Prester M, Simon MM (1986) Characterization and isolation of a trypsin-like serine protease from a long-term cultured cytotoxic T cell line by functionally distinct T cells. J Immunol 136:4644–4651

Krönke M, Leonard WJ, Depper JM, Greene WC (1985) Sequential expression of genes involved in human T lymphocyte growth and differentiation. J Exp Med 161:1593–1598

Kupfer A, Dennert G (1984) Reorientation of the microtubule-organizing center and the Golgi apparatus in cloned cytotoxic lymphocytes triggered by binding to lysable target cells. J Immunol 133:2762–2766

Lobe CG, Havele C, Bleackley RC (1986a) Cloning of two genes which are specifically expressed in activated cytotoxic T lymphocytes. Proc Natl. Acad Sci USA 83:1448–1452

Lobe CG, Finlay B, Paranchych W, Paetkau VH, Bleackley RC (1986b) Two cytotoxic T lymphocyte-specific genes encode unique serine proteases. Science 232:858–861

Lobe CG, Upton C, Duggan B, Ehrman N, Letellier M, Bell J, McFadden G, Bleackley RC (1988a) Organization of the genes encoding two T cell specific proteases, CCPI and II. Biochemistry (in press)

Lobe CG, Shaw J, Fregeau C, Meier M, Brewer A, Patient RK, Paetkau VH, Bleackley RC (1988b) Transcriptional regulation of two CTL-specific serine protease genes. (Submitted for publication)

Martz E, Heagy W, Gromkowski SH (1983) The mechanism of CTL-mediated killing: monoclonal antibody analysis of the roles of killer and target-cell membrane proteins. Immunol Rev 72:73–96

Masson D, Tschopp J (1987) A family of serine esterases in lytic granules of cytolytic T lymphocytes. Cell 49:679–685

Masson D, Nabholz M, Estrade C, Tschoop J (1986) Granules of cytolytic T-lymphocytes contain two serine esterases. EMBO J 5:1595–1600

Mills GB, Cheung RK, Grinstein S, Gelfand EW (1985a) Increase in cytosolic-free calcium concentration is an intracellular messenger for the production of interleukin 2 but not for expression of the interleukin 2 receptor. J Immunol 134:1640–1643

Mills GB, Cheung RK, Grinstein S, Gelfand EW (1985b) Interleukin 2-induced lymphocyte proliferation is independent of increases in cytosolic-free calcium concentrations. J Immunol 134:2431–2435

Milner RJ, Sutcliffe JG (1983) Gene expression in rat brain. Nucleic Acids Res 11:5497–5520

Mueller C, Gershenfeld HK, Lobe CG, Okada CY, Bleackley RC, Weissman IL (1988) A high proportion of T-lymphocytes that infiltrate H-2 incompatible heart allografts in vivo express genes encoding cytotoxic cell specific serine proteases, but do not express the MEL-14 defined lymph node homing receptor. J Exp Med 167:1124–1136

Murphy MEP, Bleackley RC, Gershenfeld HK, Weissman IL, James, MNG (1988) Comparative molecular models for two serine proteinases from cytotoxic T lymphocytes. (Submitted for publication)

Ostergaard HL, Kane KP, Mescher MF, Clarke WR (1987) Cytotoxic T lymphocyte mediated lysis without the release of serine esterases. Nature 330:71–72

Pasternack MS, Eisen HN (1985) A novel serine esterase expressed by cytotoxic T lymphocytes. Nature 314:743–745

Podack ER, Konigsberg PJ (1984) Cytolytic T cell granules. Isolation, structural, biochemical, and functional characterization. J Exp Med 160:695–710

Redelman D, Hudig D (1980) The mechanism of cell mediated cytotoxicity I. Killing by murine cytotoxic T lymphocytes requires cell surface thiols and activated proteases. J Immunol 124:870–878

Redmond MJ, Letellier M, Parker JMR, Lobe CG, Havele C, Paetkau V, Bleackley RC (1987) A serine protease (CCP1) is sequestered in the cytoplasmic granules of cytotoxic T lymphocytes. J Immunol 139:3184–3188

Reid KBM (1986) Complement-like cytotoxicity? Nature 322:684–685

Rogers J (1985) Exon shuffling and intron insertion in serine protease genes. Nature 315:458–459

Russel JH (1983) Internal disintegration model of cytotoxic lymphocyte-induced target damage. Immunol Rev 72:97–118

Shaw G, Kamen R (1986) A conserved AU sequence from the 3' untranslated region of GM-CSF mRNA mediates selective mRNA degradation. Cell 46:659–667

Shaw J, Meerovitch K, Elliott JF, Bleackley RC, Paetkau V (1987) Induction, suppression and superinduction of lymphokine mRNA in T lymphocytes. Mol Immunol 24:409–419

Simon MM, Fruth U, Simon HG, Kramer MD (1987) Evidence for the involvement of a T-cell-associated serine protease (TSP-1) in cell killing. Ann Inst Pasteur Immunol 138:309–314

Tite JP, Janeway CA (1984) Cloned helper T cells can kill B-lymphoma cells in the presence of specific antigen: Ia-restriction and cognate vs. non-cognate interactions in cytolysis. Eur J Immunol 14:878–886

Trenn G, Takayama H, Sitkovsky MV (1987) Exocytosis of cytolytic granules may not be required for target cell lysis by cytotoxic T-lymphocytes. Nature 330:72–74

Weisbrod S (1982) Active chromatin. Nature 297:289–295

Yanagi Y, Yoshikai Y, Legget K, Clark SP, Aleksander I, Mak TW (1984) A human T cell-specific cDNA clone encodes a protein having extensive homology to immunoglobulin chains. Nature 308:145–149

Yanelli JR, Sullivan JA, Mandell GL, Engelhard VH (1986) Reorientation and fusion of cytotoxic T lymphocyte granules after interaction with target cells as determined by high resolution cinematography. J Immunol 136:377–382

Young JD, Leong LG, Liu CC, Damiano A, Wall DA, Cohn ZA (1986) Isolation and characterization of a serine esterase from cytolytic T cell granules. Cell 47:183–194

A Serine Protease-Encoding Gene That Marks Activated Cytotoxic T Cells In Vivo and In Vitro

R.J. Hershberger, C. Mueller, H.K. Gershenfeld, and I.L. Weissman

1 Introduction 81
2 CTL-Specific Genes 82
3 Expression 84
4 Inconsistencies 85
5 Expression of Serine Protease Genes In Vivo 86
6 Specificity of HF Expression 87
7 Correlations with Cytotoxicity 88
8 Conclusions 90
References 90

1 Introduction

Activated cytotoxic T lymphocytes (CTLs) are presumed to be the effectors in the lysis of virally infected or transformed host cells, the mediators of graft rejection, and the potential culprits in a number of autoimmune diseases. Unfortunately, there is no marker available that specifically identifies these cells in vivo, making it difficult to prove unequivocally that CTLs are the effector cells in these immune functions. Mature T cells are usually divided into subsets on the basis of their surface phenotype: Those that express the CD8 antigen are assumed to be potential cytotoxic cells, and those that express the CD4 antigen, potential helper cells. However, the identification of $CD4^+CD8^-$ CTLs (GOLDING et al. 1985) and $CD4^-CD8^+$ helper cells (SWAIN and PANFILI 1979) both in vitro and in graft rejection in vivo (ROSENBERG et al. 1987) limits the usefulness of this division. A more serious problem with using phenotype to imply function is that these markers are expressed on both active and resting T cells. Thus, they cannot be used to distinguish between the cells participating in a localized immune response and those nonspecifically present at the site. To identify cytotoxic lymphocytes more accurately, we used a molecular genetic approach to isolate genes expressed by these cells.

Laboratory of Experimental Oncology, Department of Pathology, Stanford University School of Medicine, Stanford, CA 94305, USA

Current Topics in Microbiology and Immunology, Vol. 140
© Springer-Verlag Berlin · Heidelberg 1988

2 CTL-Specific Genes

We wanted to isolate genes expressed in CTLs that were not expressed in other cell types. To accomplish this, we created a cDNA library from the poly-A$^+$ mRNA of a murine cytotoxic T-cell line and screened it with that same RNA, labeled, in the presence of a several hundred-fold excess of unlabeled total RNA from a noncytolytic T-cell tumor (GERSHENFELD and WEISSMAN 1986). The one CTL-specific cDNA isolated was found to encode a serine protease whose sequence was homologous to human clotting factor IX, the Christmas factor; therefore, this clone was called the "Hanukah factor" (HF). Other investigators used similar approaches to identify CTL-specific genes. LOBE et al. (1986) used differential hybridization to isolate a cDNA encoding a distinct CTL serine protease named CCP1 (or C11). BRUNET et al. (1986) made a CTL minus B-cell-subtracted library and cloned out two genes named CTLA-1 and CTLA-3. These turned out to be identical to CCP1 and HF, respectively.

The deduced amino acid sequences of both HF and CCP1 are homologous to other members of the serine protease family. The catalytic site residues that define serine proteases, His-57, Asp-102, and Ser-195 (using the chymotrypsin numbering convention), are conserved in these CTL proteins, as are most of the cysteine loops and residues important for folding. MURPHY et al. (1988) took advantage of this homology to create plausible structures for HF and CCP1. They took the previously determined three-dimensional structures of bovine trypsin (HUBER et al. 1974) and rat mast cell protease II (RMCPII) (ANDERSON et al. 1978) and used them as templates for molecular model building (GREER 1981). The models of HF and CCP1 they produced can be used to predict certain structural and functional characteristics of these proteins.

The amino acid sequence of HF is homologous to both trypsin and RMCPII, with some segments being more similar to one than to the other. Thus, MURPHY et al. made a hybrid of the trypsin and RMCPII structures to be a template for the model of HF. The HF sequence differs from both trypsin and RCMPII in that it has an unpaired cysteine residue. In the HF model, the gamma sulfhydryl of the free cysteine is exposed on the surface; therefore, the model predicts that HF should form a disulfide-linked dimer. The model for CCP1 was derived from RMPCII alone, since the two are 48% similar at the amino acid level. CCP1 has a free cysteine that RMCPII lacks, but its sulfhydryl group is less exposed to the surface than that of HF. Because of this, the CCP1 model makes no clear prediction about CCP1 dimer formation.

MURPHY et al. also used these models to predict cleavage specificities for HF and CCP1. Serine proteases have a "specificity pocket": a region of the protease that binds the specific amino acid side chain of the protein to be cleaved. In the model of HF, the specificity pocket is derived from trypsin, and the conservation of an aspartic acid in the bottom of the pocket gives HF, like trypsin, a specificity for cleavage after lysine or arginine residues. The major difference between the specificity pockets of CCP1 and RCMPII is the substitution of an arginine in CCP1 for Ala-226 in RMCPII. This positive charge in the specificity pocket implies that CCP1 should cleave after an acidic aspartate or glutamate residue.

Most serine proteases are synthesized in an inactive form: they are activated when another serine protease cleaves off an initial, unconserved segment. Most serine proteases, including HF, have a lysine or arginine at the cleavage site, but CCP1 has a glutamic acid in this position. Thus the active HF protein, which cleaves after basic residues, could activate other HF molecules but not CCP1, whereas CCP1, which cleaves after acidic residues, could activate itself but not HF. If a serine protease cascade analogous to the complement or blood clotting cascade exists in CTLs, at least one more member must be involved.

The presence of serine proteases in murine CTLs was first postulated by investigators who found that some protease inhibitors could decrease target lysis (REDELMAN and HUDIG 1980; CHANG and EISEN 1980). Since then, several investigators have detected one or more proteins in activated CTLs, using either a radioactively labeled serine protease inhibitor, DFP, or an assay for trypsin-like activity (PETTY et al. 1984; PASTERNAK and EISEN 1985; MASSON et al. 1986a; KRAMER et al. 1986; YOUNG et al. 1986b). MASSON and TSCHOPP (1987) recently isolated up to eight different serine proteases from the granules of CTLs; they call these granule enzymes "granzymes." They sequenced the N-terminal 20 amino acids of these proteins, and this identified granzyme A as the protein encoded by HF (MASSON et al. 1986b). The first 20 amino acids of granzymes B, G, and H are identical, and their sequence is the same as that of CCP1. Granzyme A is a disulfide-linked homodimer with an apparent molecular weight of 60 K under nonreducing conditions and 35 K under reducing conditions (MASSON et al. 1986a). It is a functional serine protease; it cleaves synthetic peptide substrates after arginine or lysine, in agreement with the HF model. It also has an esterase activity, and its ability to cleave the synthetic ester benzyloxycarbonyl-L-lysine thiobenzyl (BLT) is the basis of a simple, colorometric assay used to detect the protein. The similarity of size, cellular location, substrate specificity, and sensitivity to inhibitors implies that granzyme A, BLT-esterase (PASTERNAK and EISEN 1985), SE-1 (YOUNG et al. 1986b), and TSP-1 (KRAMER et al. 1986) are either the HF-encoded protein or are very closely related to it. For the purposes of this review, they are all assumed to be the HF protein.

We wanted to ascertain whether human CTLs and natural killer (NK) cells also express serine protease genes. To do this, we probed a cDNA library from phytohemagglutinin-stimulated human peripheral blood leukocytes (PBL) with the mouse HF gene (GERSHENFELD et al. 1988). Only one hybridizing cDNA was found in this library, so we then used that clone to screen a human CTL library. The CTL library had a high frequency of hybridizing cDNA clones, and all those isolated had the same sequence as the first clone. In the protease-encoding domain, the sequence of the human HF (HuHF) gene is 71% and 77% similar to murine HF at the amino acid and DNA levels, respectively. All of the major structural features of the murine gene are conserved in the human homologue; thus HuHF probably also encodes a serine protease with a specificity for lysine or arginine residues. SCHMID and WEISSMANN (1987) also recently cloned a cDNA encoding a serine protease from human CTLs. It is 68% similar to CCP1 at the amino acid level and may be the homologous human gene.

The presence of a trypsin-like serine protease in human CTLs has recently been established by FERGUSON et al. (1988). They found a DFP-binding protein in cloned CTLs but not in B cells. This protein cleaves BLT, is a dimer, and has the same pattern of inhibitor sensitivity as the murine BLT esterase, suggesting that it may be the HuHF protein.

3 Expression

The murine HF gene is transcribed primarily in cytotoxic cells (GERSHENFELD and WEISSMAN 1986; BRUNET et al. 1987). Nude mouse spleens, which are enriched in natural killer cells, and a rat NK leukemia also express HF. This and the presence of lytic granules and perforin in NK cells (PODACK and DENNERT 1983; HENKART et al. 1984) suggest that the postrecognition lytic mechanisms of CTLs and NK cells may be the same. Table 1 shows that the expression of HF mRNA correlates with cytotoxicity. The HF gene hybridizes strongly with RNA from the two CTL lines, but it fails to hybridize with RNA from the noncytolytic T- and B-cell tumors tested. The HF gene also does not hybridize at a detectable level with RNA from unstimulated lymphoid tissues, such as thymus and spleen, suggesting that HF is not transcribed in nonactivated lymphocytes. Table 1 shows that HF hybridizes with RNA from eight of eight allogeneic CTL lines and from two of eight helper T-cell lines. Both of these helper lines and none of the other six had measurable cytolytic activity in a lectin-dependent, ^{51}Cr release assay.

We also examined the relative kinetics of the induction of HF mRNA and cytotoxicity (GERSHENFELD and WEISSMAN 1986). Spleen cells were stimulated in vitro with concanavalin A (Con A) and interleukin-2 (IL-2) and RNA dot blots done on samples from each day. Hybridizing RNA was undetectable at

Table 1. Expression of HF mRNA (GERSHENFELD and WEISSMAN 1986)[a]

Hybridization to poly-A$^+$ RNA (Northern analysis)		Hybridization to RNA from 5×10^5 cells (dot blots)			
		CTL clones		T-helper clones	
Thymus	–				
Spleen	–				
Kidney	–	1	+	MB2-1	+
Liver	–	2	+	MD13-5.1	–
AR1	+	3	+	M13-10	–
1E4	+	4	+	LB2-1	+
VL3	–	5	+	HDZ-9	–
L691	–	6	+	H39-34	–
RL12	–	7	+	MDK-3.5	–
M2	–	8	+	MDK-1.2	–

AR1 and *1E4*, CTL lines; *VL3*, *L691*, and *RL12*, noncytolytic T-cell tumors; *M2*, B-cell tumor line

[a] CTL lines defined by cytolysis of allogeneic targets; T-helper lines defined by lymphokine-secretion properties

the initiation of culture, was barely visible on day 2, and peaked on day 4, just preceding the appearance of cytotoxic activity in this culture.

Other investigators have tested the correlation of HF protein expression with cytotoxicity. PASTERNAK and EISEN (1985) show that the BLT-esterase is present at a much higher level in CTL clones than in noncytotoxic cells. They also note that activating thymocytes with Con A and IL-2 for 4 days causes a 100-fold increase in esterase activity. MASSON et al. (1986a) follow a more specific induction. The T-cell hybrid PC60 is not cytotoxic in the absence of growth factors, but when it is cultured with IL-1 and IL-2 it becomes cytolytically active. The BLT-esterase activity and the DFP-binding protein are induced concomitantly with cytotoxicity.

The cellular location of the HF protein supports the potential link between HF and cytotoxicity. When CTL lines are gently lysed and their subcellular components are fractionated on a Percoll gradient, the BLT-esterase activity associated with HF cosediments with the dense granule fraction (see JENNE and TSCHOPP, this volume). These isolated granules are capable of lysing erythrocytes, largely because they contain the pore-forming protein, perforin (PODACK and KONIGSBERG 1984; YOUNG and COHN 1986). When CTL clones are incubated with a serine esterase indicator substrate and morphologically examined, only the cytoplasmic granules are stained (YOUNG et al. 1986b). These granules are presumably exocytosed after a CTL binds its target (HENKART 1985; YANNELLI et al. 1986). Triggering various CTL lines with either their target (PASTERNAK et al. 1986) or T-cell receptor-specific antibodies (TAKAYAMA et al. 1987) causes the BLT-esterase to be secreted into the medium. The data presented thus far are consistent with the model that one or more serine proteases are produced during the induction of a cytotoxic cell and are secreted along with other granule components after the activated CTL binds its target.

4 Inconsistencies

The problem with this model lies in the expression of the HF protease by some noncytolytic T cells in vitro. GARCIA-SANZ et al. (1987) found that separating mouse T cells into $CD4^+CD8^-$ and $CD4^-CD8^+$ subsets and culturing them on irradiated allogeneic spleen cells for 5 days in the presence of IL-2 led to a high level of granzyme A expression in both populations. Most of the cytolytic activity and perforin, however, were in the $CD4^-CD8^+$ fraction. In contrast, DENNERT et al. (1987) showed that sensitizing T cells in vitro with fully allogeneic stimulators induced BLT-esterase and cytolytic activities, while sensitizing them with congenic stimulators differing only at the MHC class II locus caused no increase in either activity. These cultures differed from those of GARCIA-SANZ in that they contained no exogenous IL-2. SIMON et al. (1986b) also found that antigen and IL-2 could induce protease expression in both $CD4^-CD8^+$ and $CD4^+CD8^-$ populations. However, another experiment they did on unseparated T cells revealed that protease production increased with increasing amounts of IL-2. Because of this, they checked the level of protease produced by cells activated in vivo. Using immunogens chosen to stimulate either a $CD4^-CD8^+$ or $CD4^+CD8^-$ T-cell response, they discovered that the activated $CD4^-CD8^+$ cells expressed the protease while the activated $CD4^+CD8^-$ cells did not. These results suggest that nonphysiological culture conditions, in particular a high level of IL-2, may be responsible for the anomalous HF expression.

Some investigators have raised a different objection to the hypothesis that the HF serine protease is involved in cytotoxicity: the protein is not uniformly present at high levels in CTLs in vivo. The HF mRNA or protein has been found in freshly isolated $CD4^-CD8^+$ cells (SIMON et al. 1986a), peritoneal exudate lymphocytes (PEL) (BRUNET et al. 1986; MUNGER et al. 1987), and NK cells (GERSHENFELD and WEISSMAN 1986; BRUNET et al. 1986). Human NK cells ($CD3^-CD16^+$) and CTLs ($CD3^+CD16^-$) purified directly from peripheral blood express the human HF transcript (GERSHENFELD et al. 1988). However, DENNERT et al. (1987) found equally potent cytotoxicity but much less esterase activity in in vivo-stimulated PEL and NK populations than in cultured CTL lines or in vitro-activated CTLs. Also, different CTL lines can express widely varying amounts of HF (BRUNET et al. 1987).

From the above results we can draw two conclusions: the HF serine protease is not sufficient for cytotoxicity, and the level of HF expression does not necessarily correlate with cytolytic potential, especially in vitro. Neither of these rules out a requirement for HF in the cytolytic mechanism. Also, the experiments reported above do not provide absolutely reliable evidence on the specificity of HF expression. The in vitro results are suspect due to the nonphysiological culture conditions; the in vivo results suffer from the heterogeneity of the test populations. To circumvent both these problems, we have used in situ hybridization to examine the in vivo expression of the HF and CCP1 serine protease genes.

5   Expression of Serine Protease Genes In Vivo

Allograft rejections provide an excellent model for studying CTL-mediated cytolysis in vivo. We examined the expression of the serine protease genes HF and CCP1 during the rejection of myocardium grafts taken from newborn BALB/c mice ($H\text{-}2^d$) and transplanted under the kidney capsule of adult C57BL/Ka mice ($H\text{-}2^b$) (MUELLER et al. 1988). T cells are the major allograft-infiltrating cell population in this system (BILLINGHAM et al. 1977), and the allogeneic myocardium grafts are completely rejected by 8–12 days after transplantation. Using an in situ hybridization technique with radiolabeled RNA probes for either the HF or the CCP1 gene, it was demonstrated that transcripts of both genes are present in infiltrating cells as early as 2 days after transplantation (Fig. 1). The amount of protease mRNA per positive cell was initially low, but it increased constantly over the course of the graft rejection. The number of cells containing transcripts of these two genes increased dramatically between days 4 and 8 after transplantation. HF-positive cells were approximately as frequent

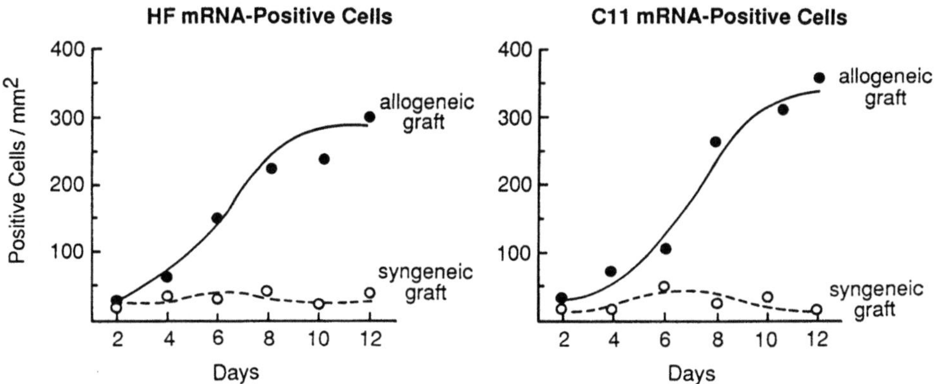

Fig. 1. Number of HF or CCP1 (here called *C11*) mRNA-positive cells per mm² infiltrate at various intervals after transplantation of heart graft

as CCP1-positive cells in the inflammatory infiltrate of the allografts, and there was no difference in the localization of both types of cells. For technical reasons we could not carry out a double labeling with both gene probes. However, our results with cloned CTLs suggest that at least some of the infiltrating cells should express both protease genes.

We also used in situ hybridizations to study the expression of HuHF, a human serine protease gene. The preliminary results indicate that this gene is expressed during cell-mediated cytolysis in humans. Using a radiolabeled RNA probe for the HuHF gene, we found HuHF mRNA-containing cells in skin lesions from patients with lichen planus and tuberculoid leprosy (C. MUELLER, G. WOOD and R. MODLIN, unpublished observations). In these experiments the amount of HuHF mRNA in the positive cells seemed to be lower than the amount of the murine transcript in the allograft experiments.

6 Specificity of HF Expression

To determine the phenotype of the HF- and CCP1-expressing cells, the allograft-infiltrating cells were sorted at 6 days after transplantation into $CD4^+CD8^-$ and $CD4^-CD8^+$ populations. The subsequent in situ hybridizations revealed that in this allograft model, HF- and CCP1-positive cells were primarily but not exclusively found among the $CD4^-CD8^+$ T cells (Fig. 2). We also checked the number and phenotype of HF- and CCP1-positive cells in the spleens of the same animals. The majority of positive cells were found in the $CD4^-CD8^+$ fraction here as well, but the fraction of that population which contained HF or CCP1 transcripts was more than ten times lower than in the allografts (Fig. 2). We found no evidence for a significant contribution of the $Thy-1^-$, $Thy-1^+CD4^-CD8^-$, or $Thy-1^+CD4^+CD8^+$ populations to the pool of HF- or CCP1-positive cells.

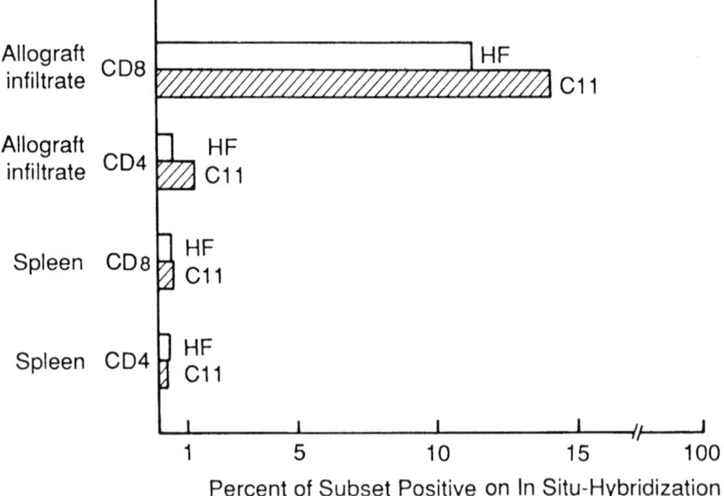

Fig. 2. Fraction of CD4$^+$CD8$^-$ and CD4$^-$CD8$^+$ T cells of the inflammatory infiltrate and the spleen expressing the HF or CCP1 gene 6 days after transplantation of an allogeneic myocardium

The in situ hybridizations of tissue sections from heart muscle allografts show that 1%–8% of the infiltrating cells express the serine protease genes by 4 or more days after transplantation. This relatively small fraction of positive cells is consistent with the observation that the majority of graft-infiltrating cells do not appear to be specific for the alloantigens of the graft (OROSZ et al. 1986; ASCHER et al. 1980). Indications that only a small fraction of the infiltrating cells in an inflammatory site may be required for cell-mediated cytolysis were recently found by SEDGWICK et al. (1987). They could induce experimental allergic encephalomyelitis in both unirradiated and irradiated rats by injecting T cells specific for myelin basic protein, even though the irradiated animals lacked the massive inflammatory infiltration of the central nervous system that was observed in the unirradiated group. Extrapolating from this, we can interpret the low level of T cells expressing the serine protease genes in an allograft as evidence that those genes are present primarily in activated cytotoxic cells. The low percentage of positive cells may also explain the finding of DENNERT et al., reported in Section 4, that CTL-containing peritoneal exudate lymphocytes had only a low level of esterase activity.

7 Correlations with Cytotoxicity

These observations on the expression of the HF and CCP1 genes do not address the issue of whether the proteases they encode actually participate in cytolysis. However, HF does fit the suppositions for a molecule involved in the lytic mechanism: (a) it is expressed by activated cytotoxic cells in vivo, (b) its expression is induced in parallel with cytotoxicity, (c) it is secreted when a CTL binds its target via its antigen receptor or when its antigen receptors are cross-linked by antibody, and (d) it is located in the same granules that, when isolated, can lyse certain targets. Since HF is not a directly lytic molecule (SIMON et al. 1986b), if it participates in cytolysis it must do so by acting on or in concert with other molecules.

The best evidence that HF may be a required participant in lytic events comes from inhibitor studies. LAVIE et al. (1985) showed that human NK-cell cytotoxicity can be blocked in a dose-dependent fashion by aprotinin, a general serine protease inhibitor, and TCPK, a chymotrypsin inhibitor. Furthermore, they found that pretreatment with aprotinin did not block cytotoxicity; sensitivity to that inhibitor existed only in the first 2 min after the effectors and targets were mixed. They concluded from this that one or more serine proteases necessary for cytotoxicity are normally sequestered, and these proteases are exposed and act just after the effector cell binds its target.

PASTERNAK and EISEN (1985) found that lysis by a cloned CTL and its BLT-esterase were inhibited by PMSF, another serine protease inhibitor. However, the concentration of PMSF that inhibited the esterase activity in the CTL lysate by 97% only decreased killing about 50%. There are several possible explanations for this. The first is that the BLT-esterase may not be involved in lysis; there may be another PMSF-sensitive molecule whose inhibition is responsible for the observed decrease. The second is that CTLs may have other mechanisms that contribute to lysis independently, such as lymphotoxin-mediated lysis (RUDDLE and SCHMID 1987) or activation of a target-cell autolytic pathway (RUSSELL et al. 1980; COHEN and DUKE 1984; UCKER 1987). In this case the PMSF-insensitive mechanisms would continue to operate, and lysis would be diminished but not eliminated. A third explanation is that the relative concentrations of protease and PMSF may be different in the effector-target contact zone than in the whole cell lysate, either because PMSF cannot easily diffuse into that zone or because the local concentration of HF is very high. A fourth possibility is that the lytic process may require only a small amount of protease activity.

One problem with drawing conclusions from the above experiments is that PMSF and aprotinin are general serine protease inhibitors rather than HF-specific inhibitors. Seven other granule proteases (MASSON and TSCHOPP 1987) and at least one surface-associated protease (UTSUNOMIYA and NAKANISHI 1986) have been found in CTLs, and their inhibition may be partially or fully responsible for the drop in lytic activity. SIMON et al. (1987) addressed this issue by using a more specific inhibitor, one based on the HF substrate most readily cleaved in their tests. Incubating intact CTL clones with this molecule did not diminish their ability to lyse their targets, but the inhibitor did block lysis by isolated granules. This finding implies that HF participates in granule-mediated lysis, since the explanations given above can account for the dichotomy between intact cells and isolated granules.

The large number of CTL serine proteases suggests that they may act in a cascade analogous to the complement or blood-clotting cascade. In these cascades, the multiple proteases act on one another in a specific order: when the first protease is activated, it cleaves and thus activates the second, and so on, until the final active product is formed. The final component of the complement cascade, C9, is functionally and antigenically similar to perforin (YOUNG et al. 1986a), which provides more circumstantial evidence for the analogy. However, there are as yet no experimental data to support or refute this hypothesis. Highly specific inhibitors will help define the function of HF and the other proteases, but to understand fully how these enzymes contribute to lymphocyte lysis, it will be necessary to determine their natural substrates and to identify the other molecules involved.

8 Conclusions

The HF gene can be a valuable tool whether or not the HF protease participates in the lytic mechanism. HF and its counterpart, CCP1, have the important distinction of being markers for activated cytotoxic lymphocytes in vivo. Thus, they can be used to evaluate the participation of cytolytic cells in various immune responses more accurately than was previously possible. More importantly, the human genes may eventually be useful for diagnosing both organ transplant rejections and some autoimmune diseases. Of course, if HF is a necessary part of the lytic mechanism and an inhibitor that works on intact cells can be found, then knowing how and when HF works will be of both therapeutic and diagnostic significance.

Acknowledgements. We thank G. Griffiths, B. Adkins, and J. Hershberger for their helpful suggestions on improving this manuscript. We gratefully acknowledge the receipt of a postdoctoral fellowship from the Swiss National Science Foundation (C.M.) and support from USPHS grants AI 19512 and OIG CA 42551. A portion of this work was supported by a grant from the Weingart Foundation.

References

Anderson WF, Matthews BW, Woodbury RG (1978) Crystallographic data for a group specific protease from rat intestine. Biochemistry 17:819

Ascher NL, Hoffman R, Chen S, Simmons RL (1980) Specific and nonspecific infiltration of sponge matrix allografts by specifically sensitized cytotoxic lymphocytes. Cell Immunol 52:38–47

Billingham M, Warnke R, Weissman IL (1977) The cellular infiltrate in cardiac allograft rejection in mice. Transplantation 23:171–176

Brunet JF, Dosseto M, Denizot F, Mattei MG, Clark WR, Haqqi TH, Ferrier P, Nabholz M, Schmitt-Verhulst AM, Luciani MF, Golstein P (1986) The inducible cytotoxic T-lymphocyte-associated gene transcript CTLA-1 sequence and gene localization to mouse chromosome 14. Nature 322:268–271

Brunet J-F, Denizot F, Suzan M, Haas W, Mencia-Huerta J-M, Berke G, Luciani M-F, Golstein P (1987) CTLA-1 and CTLA-3 serine esterase transcripts are detected mostly in cytotoxic T cells, but not only and not always. J Immunol 138:4102–4105

Chang TW, Eisen H (1980) Effects of N-tosyl-L-lysyl-chloromethylketone on the activity of cytotoxic T lymphocytes. J Immunol 124:1028–1033

Cohen JJ, Duke RC (1984) Glucocorticoid activation of a calcium-dependent endonuclease in thymocyte nuclei leads to cell death. J Immunol 132:38–42

Dennert G, Podack ER (1983) Cytolysis by H-2-specific T killer cells. Assembly of tubular complexes on target membranes. J Exp Med 157:1483–1495

Dennert G, Anderson CG, Prochazka G (1987) High activity of *N*-alpha-benzyloxycarbonyl-L-lysine thiobenzyl ester serine esterase and cytolytic perforin in cloned cell lines is not demonstrable in in-vivo-induced cytotoxic effector cells. Proc Natl Acad Sci USA 84:5004–5008

Ferguson WS, Verret CR, Reilly EB, Iannini MJ, Eisen HN (1988) Serine esterase and hemolytic activity in human cloned cytotoxic T lymphocytes. J Exp Med 167:528–540

Garcia-Sanz JA, Plaetinck G, Velotti F, Masson D, Tschopp J, MacDonald HR, Nabholz M (1987) Perforin is present only in normal activated Lyt2+ T lymphocytes and not in L3T4+ cells, but the serine protease ganzyme A is made by both subsets. EMBO J 6:933–938

Gershenfeld HK, Weissman IL (1986) Cloning of a cDNA for a T cell-specific serine protease from a cytotoxic T lymphocyte. Science 232:854–858

Gershenfeld HK, Hershberger RJ, Shows TB, Weissman IL (1988) Cloning and chromosomal assignment of a human cDNA encoding a T cell- and natural killer cell-specific, trypsin-like serine protease. Proc Natl Acad Sci USA 85:1184–1188

Golding H, Munitz TI, Singer A (1985) Characterization of antigen-specific, Ia-restricted, L3T4+ cytolytic T lymphocytes and assessment of thymic influence on their self specificity. J Exp Med 162:943–961

Greer J (1981) Comparative model building of the mammalian serine proteases. J Mol Biol 153:1027–1042

Henkart PA (1985) Mechanism of lymphocyte-mediated cytotoxicity. Annu Rev Immunol 3:31–58

Henkart PA, Millard PJ, Reynolds CW, Henkart MP (1984) Cytolytic activity of purified cytoplasmic granules from cytotoxic rat large granular lymphocyte tumors. J Exp Med 160:75–93

Huber R, Dietmar K, Bode W, Schwager P, Bartels K, Deisenhofer J, Steigemann W (1974) Structure of the complex formed by bovine trypsin and bovine pancreatic trypsin inhibitor. J Mol Biol 89:73–101

Kramer MD, Binninger L, Schirrmacher V, Moll H, Prester M, Simon MM (1986) Characterization and isolation of a trypsin-like serine protease from a long-term culture cytolytic T cell line and its expression by functionally distinct T cells. J Immunol 136:4644–4651

Lavie G, Leib Z, Servadio C (1985) The mechanism of human NK-cell-mediated cytotoxicity. Mode of action of surface-associated proteases in the early stages of the lytic reaction. J Immunol 135:1470–1476

Lobe CG, Finlay BB, Paranchych W, Paetkau VH, Bleackley RC (1986) Novel serine proteases encoded by two cytotoxic T lymphocyte-specific genes. Science 232:858–861

Masson D, Tschopp J (1987) A family of serine esterases in lytic granules of cytolytic T lymphocytes. Cell 49:679–685

Masson D, Nabholz M, Estrade C, Tschopp J (1986a) Granules of cytolytic T-lymphocytes contain two serine esterases. EMBO J 5:1595–1600

Masson D, Zamai M, Tschopp J (1986b) Identification of granzyme A isolated from cytotoxic T-lymphocyte-granules as one of the proteases encoded by CTL-specific genes. FEBS Lett 208:84–88

Mueller C, Gershenfeld HK, Lobe CG, Okada CY, Bleackley RC, Weissman IL (1988) A high proportion of T-lymphocytes that infiltrate H-2 incompatible heart allografts in vivo express genes encoding cytotoxic, cell-specific serine proteases, but do not express the MEL-14 defined lymph node-homing receptor. J Exp Med 167:1124–1136

Munger WE, Berrebi G, Henkart PA (1987) Granule exocytosis by cytotoxic T lymphocytes generated in vivo. Ann Inst Pasteur Immunol 138:301–304

Murphy MEP, Bleackley RC, Gershenfeld HK, Weissman IL, James MNG (1988) Comparative molecular models for two serine proteinases from cytotoxic T lymphocytes. (manuscript in preparation)

Orosz CG, Zinn NE, Sirinek L, Ferguson RM (1986) In vivo mechanisms of alloreactivity 1. Frequency of donor-reactive, cytotoxic T-lymphocytes in sponge matrix allografts. Transplantation 41:75–83

Pasternack MS, Eisen HN (1985) A novel serine esterase expressed by cytotoxic T lymphocytes. Nature 314:743–745

Pasternack MS, Verret CR, Liu MA, Eisen HN (1986) Serine esterase in cytolytic T lymphocytes. Nature 322:740–743

Petty HR, Hermann W, Dereski W, Frey T, McConnell H (1984) Activatable esterase activity of murine natural killer cell-YAC tumor cell conjugates. J Cell Sci 72:1–13

Podack ER, Dennert G (1983) Assembly of two types of tubules with putative cytolytic function by cloned natural killer cells. Nature 302:442–445

Podack ER, Konigsberg PJ (1984) Cytolytic T cell granules. Isolation, structural, biochemical, and functional characterization. J Exp Med 160:695–710

Redelman D, Hudig D (1980) The mechanism of cell mediated cytotoxicity I. Killing by murine cytotoxic T lymphocytes requires cell surface thiols and activated proteases. J Immunol 124:870–878

Rosenberg AS, Mizuochi T, Sharrow SO, Singer A (1987) Phenotype, specificity, and function of T cell subsets and T cell interactions involved in skin allograft rejection. J Exp Med 165:1296–1315

Ruddle NH, Schmid DS (1987) The role of lymphotoxin in T-cell-mediated cytotoxicity. Ann Inst Pasteur Immunol 138:314–320

Russell JH, Masakowski VR, Dobos CB (1980) Mechanisms of immune lysis. I. Physiological distinction between target cell death mediated by cytotoxic T lymphocytes and antibody plus complement. J Immunol 124:1100–1105

Schmid J, Weissmann C (1987) Induction of mRNA for a serine protease and a beta-thromboglobulin-like protein in mitogen-stimulated human leukocytes. J Immunol 139:250–256

Sedgwick J, Brostoff S, Mason D (1987) Experimental allergic encephalomyelitis in the absence of a classical delayed-type hypersensitivity reaction. J Exp Med 165:1058–1075

Simon MM, Hoschutzky H, Fruth U, Simon HG, Kramer MD (1986a) Purification and characterization of a T cell specific serine proteinase (TSP-1) from cloned cytolytic T lymphocytes. EMBO J 5:3267–3274

Simon MM, Fruth U, Simon HG, Kramer MD (1986b) A specific serine proteinase is inducible in Lyt-2+, L3T4− and Lyt-2−, L3T4+ T cells in vitro but is mainly associated with Lyt-2+, L3T4-effector cells in vivo. Eur J Immunol 16:1559–1568

Simon MM, Fruth U, Simon HG, Kramer MD (1987) Evidence for the involvement of a T-cell-associated serine protease (TSP-1) in cell killing. Ann Inst Pasteur Immunol 138:309–314

Swain SL, Panfili PR (1979) Helper cells activated by allogeneic H-2K or H-2D differences have a Ly phenotype distinct from those responsive to I differences. J Immunol 122:383–391

Takayama H, Trenn G, Humphrey W, Bluestone JA, Henkart PA, Sitkovsky MV (1987) Antigen receptor-triggered secretion of a trypsin-type esterase from cytotoxic T lymphocytes. J Immunol 138:566–569

Ucker DS (1987) Cytotoxic T lymphocytes and glucocorticoids activate an endogenous suicide process in target cells. Nature 327:62–64

Utsunomiya N, Nakanishi M (1986) A serine protease triggers the initial step of transmembrane signalling in cytotoxic T cells. J Biol Chem 261:16514–16517

Yannelli JR, Sullivan JA, Mandell GL, Engelhard VH (1986) Reorientation and fusion of cytotoxic T lymphocyte granules after interaction with target cells as determined by high resolution cinemicrography. J Immunol 136:377–382

Young JD, Cohn ZA (1986) Role of granule proteins in lymphocyte-mediated killing. J Cell Biochem 32:151–167

Young JD, Leong LG, Liu CC, Damiano A, Wall DA, Cohn ZA (1986b) Isolation and characterization of a serine esterase from cytolytic T cell granules. Cell 47:183–194

Young JD-E, Cohn ZA, Podack ER (1986a) The ninth component of complement and the pore-forming protein (perforin 1) from cytotoxic T cells: structural, immunological, and functional similarities. Science 233:184–190

Structure and Function of the Family of Proteoglycans That Reside in the Secretory Granules of Natural Killer Cells and Other Effector Cells of the Immune Response

R.L. Stevens, M.M. Kamada, and W.E. Serafin

1   Introduction 93
2   Proteoglycan Biochemistry 94
3   Mast Cell Secretory Granule Proteoglycans 96
3.1 Identification, Distribution, and Structure 96
3.2 Molecular Biology of Secretory Granule Proteoglycans 97
3.3 Interaction of Secretory Granule Proteoglycans with Proteases 100
4   Proteoglycans in Natural Killer Cells and Large Granular Lymphocytes 102
4.1 Identification, Distribution, and Structure 102
4.2 Interaction of Natural Killer Cell Serine Proteases with Proteoglycans 103
References 105

1 Introduction

Although it has been known for a number of years that many of the effector cells that participate in immune responses have cell-associated proteoglycans, it has only recently become apparent that these highly acidic macromolecules reside within intracellular secretory granules rather than on the plasma membrane. Heparin proteoglycans are found in the secretory granules of connective tissue mast cells (CTMC) (BENDITT et al. 1956; YURT et al. 1977a, b; ROBINSON et al. 1978; METCALFE et al. 1979, 1980a; RAZIN et al. 1982; BLAND et al. 1982). Chondroitin sulfate proteoglycans are found in the secretory granules of mucosal mast cells (MMC) (STEVENS et al. 1986), lung mast cells (STEVENS et al. 1988a), basophils (ORENSTEIN et al. 1978; ROTHENBERG et al. 1987), eosinophils (MET-CALFE et al. 1982), neutrophils (OLSSON 1969; OHHASHI et al. 1984), monocytes/macrophages (LEVITT and HO 1983; KOLSET et al. 1984), HL-60 promyelocytic cells (LUIKART et al. 1984), bone marrow-derived mast cells (BMMC) (RAZIN et al. 1982; STEVENS et al. 1985), and rat basophilic leukemia-1 (RBL-1) cells (METCALFE et al. 1980b; SELDIN et al. 1985). Human (MACDERMOTT et al. 1985) and mouse (DVORAK et al. 1983) natural killer (NK) cells and rat large granular

From the Department of Medicine, Harvard Medical School; and the Department of Rheumatology and Immunology, Brigham and Women's Hospital, Boston, Mass. 02115, USA.
This work was supported in part by grants AI-23483, AI-22531, AI-23401, and HL-36110 from the National Institutes of Health. R.L.S. is an Established Investigator for the American Heart Association. W.E.S. is supported by grants from the Irvington House and the Arthritis Foundation. M.M.K. is a trainee on grant T32 AI-07306

lymphocyte (LGL) tumor cells (STEVENS et al. 1987) synthesize cell-associated chondroitin sulfate proteoglycans that are stored in cytolytic secretory granules. Because these proteoglycans are exocytosed when the effector cell kills tumor target cells (SCHMIDT et al. 1985), it has been postulated that they play a role in cell-mediated cytotoxicity. In this chapter, we will provide a brief general description of proteoglycans. It will become apparent that the secretory granule proteoglycans that reside in NK cells are very homologous to those that reside in other effector cells of the immune response. In order to understand the structure and function of NK cell proteoglycans, we will discuss in detail the more thoroughly characterized homologous proteoglycans that reside in the secretory granules of mast cells. Evidence for an ionic interaction between these acidically charged proteoglycans and basically charged endopeptidases and exopeptidases will be presented. Finally, we will review the literature concerning the role of proteoglycans in lymphocyte-mediated cytotoxicity.

2   Proteoglycan Biochemistry

All proteoglycans contain a peptide core to which one or more glycosaminoglycan side chains are attached. Because proteoglycans are the most extensively posttranslationally modified proteins in the body, they are often large macromolecules. Depending on the cell type, proteoglycan molecular weights can range from 60 K to 4000 K. The amino acid sequence of the peptide core dictates the number of N-linked, high-mannose-type oligosaccharides that are added onto the peptide core in the endoplasmic reticulum, and the number of glycosaminoglycan side chains that are polymerized in the Golgi. All heparin, heparan sulfate, and chondroitin sulfate proteoglycans have peptide cores that contain at least one Ser-Gly sequence to which a glycosaminoglycan side chain is attached via an O-glycosic linkage (MUIR 1958; LINDAHL et al. 1965; ISEMURA and IKENAKA 1975). Recent studies have indicated that peptide cores of proteoglycans have one or two acidic amino acids preceding the first glycosylated Ser-Gly sequence (BOURDON et al. 1987a). During the biosynthesis of chondroitin sulfate and heparin glycosaminoglycans, sequential glycosyltransferases add UDP-monosaccharides to the peptide core, resulting in the sequence Ser → Xyl → Gal → Gal → GlcUA (see RODÉN 1980, for review). For unknown reasons, different types of cells then polymerize different types of glycosaminoglycans onto the GlcUA. These are either chondroitin sulfate glycosaminoglycan chains composed of large numbers (up to 100) of repeating GalNAc → GlcUA disaccharides or heparin/heparan sulfate glycosaminoglycan chains composed of repeating GlcNAc → GlcUA disaccharides (Fig. 1). A number of modification events then take place in the *trans* region of the Golgi to sulfate the precursor glycosaminoglycan side chain. The eventual glycosaminoglycan of 8 K–100 K that is synthesized onto the peptide core contains 1–3 sulfate groups and one carboxylic acid residue per disaccharide. The large number of sulfate and carboxylic acid residues gives proteoglycans their highly acidic charge, and as such they can tightly bind cations and basically charged proteins. Because the posttranslational events that take place during the biosynthesis of proteoglycans

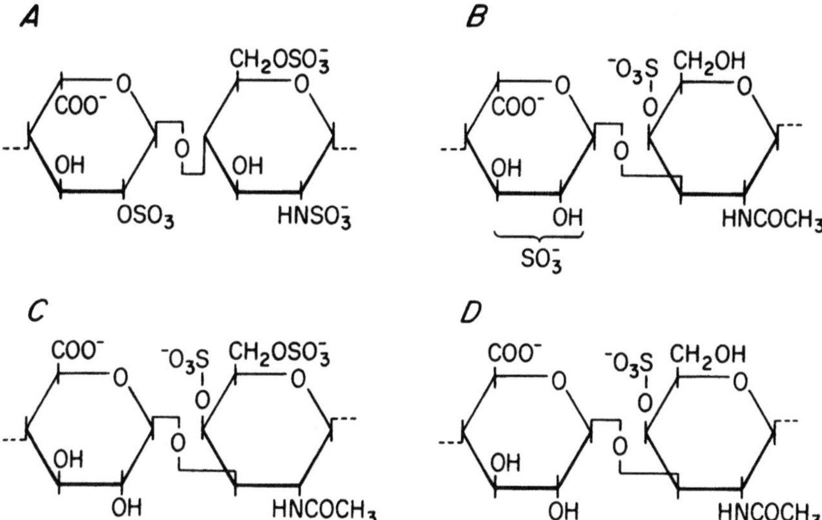

Fig. 1A–D. Structures of the major disaccharide that is repeated in CTMC heparin proteoglycan (**A**), MMC chondroitin sulfate di-B proteoglycan (**B**), BMMC chondroitin sulfate E proteoglycan (**C**), and NK cell chondroitin sulfate A proteoglycan (**D**)

are large in number and are under enzymatic control, one cell does not often produce two identical molecules. The glycosaminoglycans bound to proteoglycans can be heterogeneous in their extent of sulfation, position of sulfation, extent of phosphorylation of Xyl, extent of epimerization of GlcUA to IdUA, length, and number per peptide core. Varied Ser/Thr phosphorylation and intracellular degradation of the peptide core, and varied degrees of modification of N-linked and O-linked glycans also contribute to proteoglycan heterogeneity.

The final location of proteoglycans has been one criterion for classifying these macromolecules into subfamilies. It is now known that at least twelve distinct genes encode proteoglycan peptide cores. Many of these genes encode proteoglycans that are destined to reside in the extracellular matrix of such connective tissues as cartilage (OLDBERG et al. 1987) and skin (KRUSIUS and RUOSLAHTI 1986). Those genes that encode proteoglycans that have a hydrophobic domain in their peptide cores, such as the invariant chain proteoglycan (CLAESSON et al. 1983; GIACOLETTO et al. 1986), are destined to reside on the plasma membrane with their glycosaminoglycan side chains facing outside the cell. Genes that encode Ser-Gly-rich proteoglycan peptide cores appear to be destined to be stored inside cells within secretory granules (TANTRAVAHI et al. 1986; AVRAHAM et al. 1988; STEVENS et al. 1988b). While the proteoglycans that are found in the secretory granules of effector cells (Table 1) share some of the same basic structural features of extracellular- and pericellular-localized proteoglycans, they are clearly distinct in that they are highly resistant to degradation by such general proteases as trypsin, chymotrypsin, pronase, collagenase, pepsin, and papain (HORNER 1971; YURT et al. 1977a; STEVENS et al. 1985; SELDIN et al. 1985; MacDERMOTT et al. 1985).

Table 1. Proteoglycans and proteases of cells of the immune system

Cell type	Species	Proteoglycan	Molecular weight (K)	Protease type	pI
CTMC	rat	heparin	750	chymotryptic	9.5
MMC	rat	ChS di-B	150	chymotryptic	~8
BMMC	mouse	ChS E	200	serine	9.1
Mast cell	human	heparin	60–200	tryptic	basic
Basophil	human	ChS E/heparin	140	ND	ND
NK cell	human	ChS A	200	chymotryptic	basic
LGL	rat	ChS A	500[a]	tryptic	ND
CTL	mouse	ND	ND	tryptic	>10
NK	mouse	ChS A	ND	tryptic	ND

ND, not determined

[a] The 500 K proteoglycan is degraded and stored in the secretory granules as 85 K glycosaminoglycans (STEVENS et al. 1987)

3 Mast Cell Secretory Granule Proteoglycans

3.1 Identification, Distribution, and Structure

Mast cells were first discovered by PAUL EHRLICH (1878) over 100 years ago when he noted that there were cells in connective tissue that contained large numbers of granules which were metachromatic when stained with the cationic dye toluidine blue. Subsequent histochemical studies using other cationic dyes revealed that two general subclasses of mast cells exist in rats and mice (ENERBÄCK 1966). When stained, the secretory granules of rat MMC (located in the gastrointestinal tract mucosa) are alcian blue$^+$/safranin$^-$, while those in rat CTMC (located in the skin and peritoneal cavity) are alcian blue$^+$/safranin$^+$. These early histochemical studies indicated that different populations of rodent mast cells contained different types of acidic macromolecules packaged in their secretory granules. We now know that rat CTMC are rich in heparin proteoglycans (YURT et al. 1977a) and MMC are rich in chondroitin sulfate di-B/E proteoglycans (STEVENS et al. 1986). Depending on the species and the tissue source, the concentration of heparin proteoglycan can range from barely detectable amounts to approximately 25 pg/cell. Until recently, a controversy existed as to whether the cell-associated proteoglycans produced by mast cells resided within the secretory granules or resided on the cell surface. Different methods have been used to establish conclusively the secretory granule location of the mast cell proteoglycans. YURT and coworkers (1977b) established that there was parallel exocytosis of histamine (a secretory granule marker) and ^{35}S-labeled heparin proteoglycans from immunologically activated, ^{35}S-labeled, rat CTMC. Using a combination of electron microscopy and X-ray dispersion spectroscopy, CAULFIELD et al. (1986) demonstrated that the secretory granules of rat CTMC were the only cellular compartments that contained significant amounts of sulfur.

When incubated with cationic dyes, mast cells stain dramatically because their proteoglycans are more sulfated than the proteoglycans produced by other cells. Heparin proteoglycan is the most acidic macromolecule in the body; in the rat, it contains as many as 3000 sulfate and 1000 carboxylic acid groups per molecule. The heparin proteoglycan isolated from rat CTMC ranges from 750 K to 1000 K (ROBINSON et al. 1978; YURT et al. 1977a). It contains a small peptide core to which approximately seven 75 K–100 K heparin glycosaminoglycans are attached. The major disaccharide that is repeated within heparin is $IdUA\text{-}2SO_4 \rightarrow GlcNSO_4\text{-}6SO_4$ (Fig. 1). Rat MMC chondroitin sulfate di-B proteoglycans (STEVENS et al. 1986), mouse BMMC chondroitin sulfate E proteoglycans (RAZIN et al. 1982; STEVENS et al. 1985), human basophilic leukocyte chondroitin sulfate E proteoglycans (ROTHENBERG et al. 1987), and human lung mast cell chondroitin sulfate E proteoglycans (STEVENS et al. 1988a) are the next most acidic macromolecules in the body. These chondroitin sulfate proteoglycans range from 100 K to 250 K, have small peptide cores, and contain approximately seven 10 K–25 K chondroitin sulfate side chains. As assessed by high performance liquid chromatography (SELDIN et al. 1984), the major disaccharide that is repeated within chondroitin sulfate di-B proteoglycans and chondroitin sulfate E proteoglycans is $IdUA\text{-}2SO_4 \rightarrow GalNAc\text{-}4SO_4$ and $GlcUA \rightarrow GalNAc\text{-}4,6diSO_4$, respectively (Fig. 1). The most likely reason for their lack of safranin staining is that the major proteoglycan present in MMC and BMMC has one less sulfate residue per disaccharide than CTMC heparin proteoglycan.

The amino acid composition of the heparin proteoglycan core peptide [whether isolated from pronase-treated rat skin (ROBINSON et al. 1978) or from sonicated rat CTMC (METCALFE et al. 1980a)] has been determined. Surprisingly, the peptide core of this proteoglycan consists almost entirely of equal amounts of serine and glycine. Because heparin glycosaminoglycans were known to be linked to serines at serine-glycine sequences, it was postulated that the peptide core of rat mast cell heparin proteoglycan was predominately an alternating sequence of serine and glycine. The amino acid compositions of RBL-1 cell-derived chondroitin sulfate di-B proteoglycan (SELDIN et al. 1985) and mouse BMMC-derived chondroitin sulfate E proteoglycan peptide cores (STEVENS et al. 1985) differed from heparin proteoglycan in that substantial amounts of other amino acids (particularly glutamic acid) were detected. Because of these differences in amino acid composition, it could not be determined whether the genes that encode the peptide cores of different secretory granule-localized proteoglycans were the same or different.

3.2 Molecular Biology of Secretory Granule Proteoglycans

While the above characterization studies were being carried out on mast cell proteoglycans, OLDBERG and coworkers (1981) independently isolated and characterized an unusual proteoglycan from rat L2 yolk sac tumor cells. The *N*-terminal amino acid sequence was determined and an oligonucleotide probe made to obtain the partial cDNA (designated pPG-1) from a rat L2 cell-derived cDNA library (BOURDON et al. 1985). The deduced amino acid sequence of this and another (BOURDON et al. 1986) cDNA revealed that the corresponding

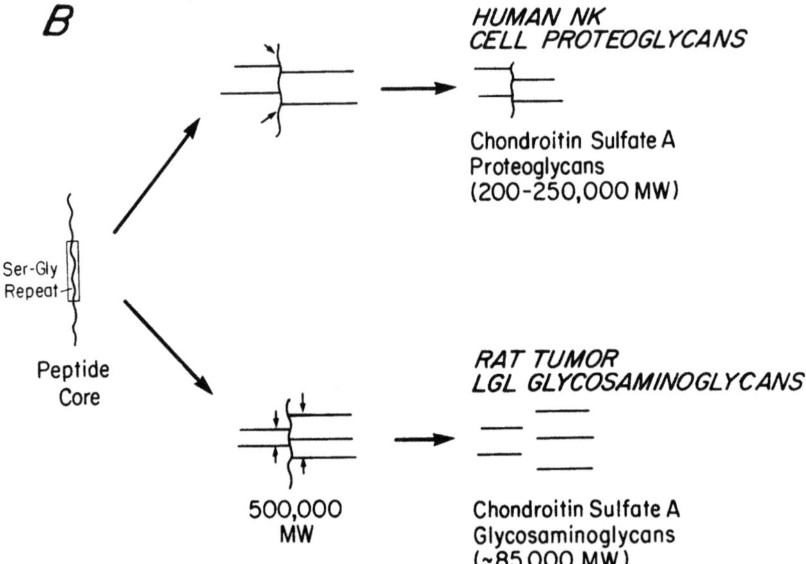

Fig. 2. A Amino acid sequence of the peptide core of the secretory granule-localized proteoglycan of rat L2 cells, mast cells, and probably LGL. The *underlined amino acids* indicate the hydrophobic signal peptide. **B** Schematic post-translation modification and degradation of the peptide core in human NK cells and rat LGL tumor cells. In human NK cells, the peptide core is presumably degraded in the secretory granule at its N- and C-terminus, leaving a glycosaminoglycan attachment region that consists primarily of alternating serine and glycine. Attached to the protein core are approximately four, 50 K, unbranched chondroitin sulfate A glycosaminoglycans, resulting in an overall molecular weight of approximately 200 K. In rat LGL tumor cells, the peptide core is presumably degraded in the secretory granule by an endoglycosidase, resulting in the storage of approximately 85 K chondroitin sulfate A glycosaminoglycans

mRNA in rat L2 cells encodes an 18.6 K proteoglycan peptide core that contains a 49 amino acid glycosaminoglycan attachment region of alternating serines and glycines (Fig. 2A). Because of this finding, these investigators proposed that the proteoglycan peptide core that is expressed in the rat L2 yolk sac tumor cell is related to the peptide core of heparin proteoglycan.

When Southern blots of rat genomic DNA were probed with pPG-1 under conditions of high stringency, the rat probe hybridized to a multigene family

(TANTRAVAHI et al. 1986; BOURDON et al. 1987b). In order to determine the relationship of the L2 cell proteoglycan peptide core to that expressed in different populations of mast cells, a gene-specific, $\sim$500-bp, SspI $\rightarrow$ 3' fragment of pPG-1 (designated pPG-M) was obtained (TANTRAVAHI et al. 1986). Using pPG-M under conditions of high stringency, it was determined that, unlike fibroblasts, all populations of rat and mouse mast cells contained substantial amounts of an approximately 1.3-kb species of mRNA that hybridized to this probe. This mRNA was present regardless of whether the cells were synthesizing heparin proteoglycans, chondroitin sulfate di-B proteoglycans, or chondroitin sulfate E proteoglycans. We concluded that the same gene was used by different populations of mast cells (and probably other effector cells) to encode the peptide core that was expressed in rat L2 yolk sac tumor cells. It remained to be determined whether or not the differences in amino acid compositions of these proteoglycan peptide cores result from different exon splicing of RNA or from different intracellular posttranslational degradation.

Recently, a cDNA that encodes the proteoglycan peptide core in RBL-1 cells was isolated from a RBL-1 cell-derived cDNA library (AVRAHAM et al. 1988). Based on the consensus nucleotide sequence and deduced amino acid sequence of this cDNA (Fig. 2A), it was determined that the translated proteoglycan peptide core in the RBL-1 cell is identical to that expressed in rat L2 yolk sac tumor cells. This finding indicated that RBL-1 cells (and therefore probably BMMC and CTMC) do not differently splice the mRNA that encodes their respective proteoglycan peptide cores. A close inspection of the deduced amino acid sequence of the RBL-1 cell proteoglycan peptide core revealed relatively high levels of glutamic acid at the C-terminus. Thus, if the same proteoglycan core peptide gene was expressed in the different populations of mast cells, the core peptide in CTMC proteoglycan must be more degraded than those in RBL-1 cells and mouse BMMC. Since RBL-1 cells and mouse BMMC have substantially less carboxypeptidase A packaged in their secretory granules than CTMC (SERAFIN et al. 1987), we concluded that the C-terminal amino acids of the heparin proteoglycan peptide core might be removed in the secretory granule when the proteoglycan interacts with this exopeptidase. The deduced amino acid sequence of the RBL-1 cell proteoglycan peptide core also revealed a 49-amino acid region composed of alternating serines and glycines (AVRAHAM et al. 1988). Since no other amino acids are present in this glycosaminoglycan attachment region, the overall molecular weight of the proteoglycan can not be substantially altered when the proteoglycan is incubated with proteolytic enzymes.

The HL-60 cells line is derived from a human promyelocytic leukemia. By using the rat probe to screen an HL-60 cell-derived cDNA library under conditions of low stringency, we isolated a cDNA that encodes the human analogue of the rat secretory granule proteoglycan core peptide (STEVENS et al. 1988b). The deduced amino acid sequence of the cDNA revealed that the molecular weight of this human proteoglycan peptide core is 17.6 K. Although the peptide core contains a serine-glycine repeat region, the region consists of only 18 amino acids, and one of the serine residues in the sequence has been replaced by a phenylalanine. While 48% of the amino acids in the rat and human proteoglycan peptide core sequences are identical, the *N*-terminus in particular is highly conserved, suggesting that this region of the peptide core is of critical importance for the biosynthesis, subcellular targeting, and/or function of these proteoglycans. Based on the analysis of different somatic cell hybrids, it was concluded that the gene that encodes this proteoglycan peptide core resides on chromosome 10 in the mouse (AVRAHAM et al. 1988) and in the human (STEVENS et al. 1988 b).

3.3 Interaction of Secretory Granule Proteoglycans with Proteases

In order to postulate what the functions of secretory granule proteoglycans might be, it is necessary to understand the properties of the other proteins that are stored in this intracellular compartment. The secretory granules of mast cells contain large amounts of basically charged proteases that are enzymatically active at neutral to basic pH. Each rat serosal CTMC contains approximately 25 pg of rat mast cell protease I (RMCP-I; also known as chymase because of its chymotrypsin-like substrate specificity) (LAGUNOFF and PRITZL 1976) and approximately 20 pg of carboxypeptidase A (EVERITT and NEURATH 1980; SERAFIN et al. 1987). Each rat MMC contains substantial amounts of a distinct chymotryptic endopeptidase which has been termed RMCP-II (WOODBURY and NEURATH 1978; BENFEY et al. 1987), while each mouse BMMC contains approximately 2 pg of a serine protease of undefined specificity (DUBUSKE et al. 1984). The isoelectric points of RMCP-I, carboxypeptidase A, RMCP-II, and the mouse BMMC serine protease are 9.5, approximately 11, approximately 8, and 9.1, respectively. Human lung mast cells contain a trypsin-like endopeptidase that also appears to possess a basic isoelectric point (SMITH et al. 1984). Because the proteoglycans and proteases are oppositely charged at the intragranular pH of 5.5, they are stored in the secretory granules ionically bound to each other. Considering that each of these secretory granule proteases is known to be stored in active form rather than as a zymogen, one of the functions of the secretory granule proteoglycans may be to package the proteases in a configuration that minimizes autolysis of the enzymes or degradation of other cellular components. Furthermore, such packaging might serve to allow a higher density of packaging of the proteases within the secretory granules.

A number of activation-secretion experiments carried out on different populations of mast cells have revealed that secretory granule proteoglycans not only interact with proteases inside the cell but also outside the cell. Because of their different isoelectric points, the protease/proteoglycan ionic complexes from rat CTMC (YURT and AUSTEN 1977c; EVERITT and NEURATH 1980; SCHWARTZ et al. 1981), mouse BMMC (SERAFIN et al. 1986, 1987), and human lung mast cells (SCHWARTZ and BRADFORD 1986) remain intact following their exocytosis from immunologically activated cells. The proteases in mouse BMMC serve to illustrate this point. Utilizing [^{3}H]diisopropyl-fluorophosphate (DFP) to radiolabel the serine proteases, it was established that the majority of the endopeptidases in the secretory granules of mouse BMMC were approximately 30 K when analyzed by sodium dodecyl sulfate polyacrylamide gel electrophoresis (DUBUSKE et al. 1984). Despite their small size, it was discovered that when

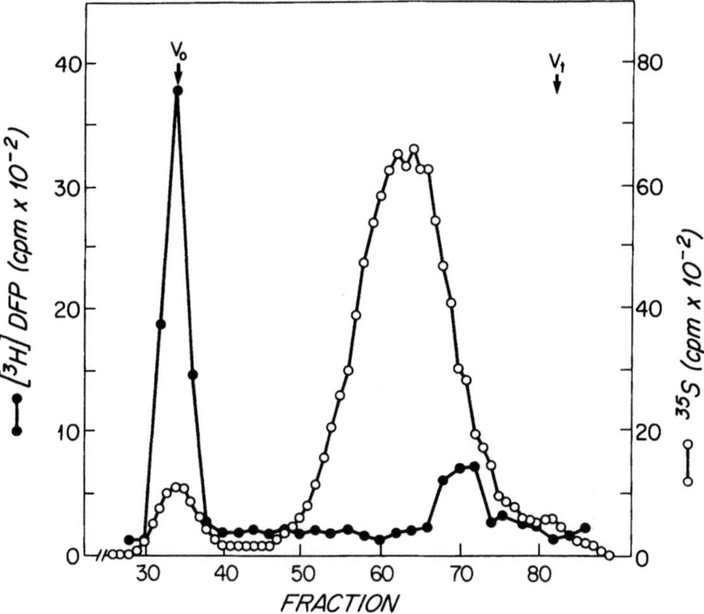

Fig. 3. Sepharose CL-2B gel filtration chromatography of [^{3}H]DFP-binding proteases (*solid circles*) and ^{35}S-labeled proteoglycans (*open circles*) exocytosed from activated mouse bone marrow-derived mast cells (from SERAFIN et al. 1986). The void volume of the column (V_0) is indicated and corresponds to a molecular weight of greater than 10000 K. More than 80% of the exocytosed serine proteases are located in a macromolecular complex with a minority of the proteoglycans. By SDS-PAGE, the molecular weight of these same serine proteases are approximately 30 K (DuBUSKE et al. 1984)

the supernatants from activated BMMC were filtered on a column of Sepharose CL-2B, the serine proteases filtered as if their molecular weights were >10 million (SERAFIN et al. 1986) (Fig. 3). This complex could be disrupted in the presence of high ionic strength buffers indicating that the proteases were ionically bound to an acidic macromolecule. When the column fractions were examined for ^{35}S-labeled proteoglycans, it was discovered that approximately 200 K chondroitin sulfate E proteoglycans and approximately 200 K heparin proteoglycans were present in approximately equal amounts in the macromolecular complex.

While the significance for macromolecular protease/proteoglycan complexes has not been fully explored, it is likely that the binding of endopeptidases and exopeptidases to a common proteoglycan molecule will influence the substrate specificity of these two types of enzymes and influence their ability to degrade common protein substrates sequentially. For example, when RMCP-I is bound to heparin proteoglycan, its ability to degrade large molecular weight protein substrates is substantially diminished (TRONG et al. 1987). The substrate specificity of RMCP-I, as defined by preferred amino acid sites for cleavage, is also altered when it is bound to heparin proteoglycan (TRONG et al. 1987).

Another predicted consequence of the continued maintenance of the proteoglycan/protease macromolecular complexes outside the cell would be to localize these enzymes in the immediate area around the activated effector cell. Mast cell proteases that have been dissociated from their proteoglycan can degrade connective tissue proteins such as type IV collagen (SAGE et al. 1979) and fibronectin (VARTIO et al. 1981; DuBUSKE et al. 1984). Thus, it is an evolutionary advantage to have a mechanism whereby proteases that are enzymatically active at neutral pH are prevented from random diffusion into other areas of connective tissue where they could do damage to the extracellular matrix.

Another important advantage of binding of the proteases to the proteoglycans is the preservation of proteolytic activity for extended periods of time. Like trypsin that is cross-linked to Sepharose, the interaction of one protease molecule with another is sterically prevented when they are both bound to proteoglycans. Autolysis is thereby minimized. In studies done with the human mast cell tryptase, SCHWARTZ and BRADFORD (1986) found that the tetrameric form of the enzyme rapidly dissociated into inactive subunits at 37° C when the enzyme was incubated in the absence of heparin. However, the enzyme was active for hours when incubated in the presence of heparin.

4 Proteoglycans in Natural Killer Cells and Large Granular Lymphocytes

4.1 Identification, Distribution, and Structure

Human peripheral blood T-lymphocytes (LEVITT and HO 1983) and mouse NK cells (DVORAK et al. 1983) have been shown to synthesize chondroitin sulfate proteoglycans. Based on the ultrastructural distribution of radiolabeled macromolecules, these chondroitin sulfate proteoglycans were tentatively localized to the secretory granules (DVORAK et al. 1983). In subsequent studies, it was shown that cloned human NK cells (MACDERMOTT et al. 1985) and purified human LGL (PARMLEY et al. 1985) possess cell-associated chondroitin sulfate proteoglycans. Because these proteoglycans were not accessible to digestion when intact NK cells were incubated with chondroitinase ABC (MACDERMOTT et al. 1985), the proteoglycans were thought to be located in an intracellular compartment rather than on the plasma membrane of the cell. The demonstration by X-ray microanalysis that the electron dense secretory granules of the human NK cell were rich in sulfur-containing macromolecules was conclusive evidence that these chondroitin sulfate proteoglycans were stored there (MACDERMOTT et al. 1985). As assessed by high performance liquid chromatography of chondroitinase ABC digests, the NK cell-derived proteoglycans were different from the mast cell-derived proteoglycans in that they were less sulfated. Chondroitin sulfate A appears to be the only glycosaminoglycan bound to NK cell proteoglycans (Fig. 1). The first clear evidence that the peptide cores of the proteoglycans that are stored in the secretory granules of NK cells are very homologous to those stored in mast cells was that their macromolecules are also resistant to proteolytic degradation (MACDERMOTT et al. 1985).

Because large numbers of cells can be obtained per animal, tumors of rat LGL have been valuable for characterizing the molecules packaged in cytolytic secretory granules (REYNOLDS et al. 1984). Like human NK cells, rat LGL tumor cells synthesize protease-resistant chondroitin sulfate A proteoglycans (STEVENS et al. 1987). The difference between rat LGL tumor cells and normal human NK cells is that the 500 K proteoglycans in the former are metabolized intracellularly to individual 85 K glycosaminoglycans. When enriched by Percoll density gradient centrifugation, it was discovered that the cytolytic secretory granules contain predominately chondroitin sulfate A glycosaminoglycan side chains rather than intact chondroitin sulfate A proteoglycans (STEVENS et al. 1987). Since heparin proteoglycans are also metabolized inside transformed mast cells to individual glycosaminoglycans (OGREN and LINDAHL 1975), the presence of these chondroitin sulfate A glycosaminoglycans in the granules of LGL tumor cells is probably a consequence of the transformed nature of these cells rather than a species difference. The discovery that these rat LGL contain an approximate 1.3-kb species of mRNA that hybridizes under conditions of high stringency to pPG-1 and pPG-M (STEVENS et al. 1987) indicates that the same rat gene encoding the CTMC-derived heparin proteoglycan peptide core (TANTRAVAHI et al. 1986) also encodes the LGL-derived chondroitin sulfate A proteoglycan peptide core. This finding raises the interesting possibility that rat L2 cells are tumor cells because they aberrantly synthesize and constitutively exocytose a proteoglycan that is normally only expressed in NK cells and other effector cells. It remains to be determined whether the HL-60 cell secretory granule proteoglycan peptide core is also expressed in human NK cells.

Human NK cells specifically exocytose their secretory granule proteoglycans when they kill tumor cells (MACDERMOTT et al. 1985). As expected for release of a granule constituent, the extent of release of proteoglycan is dependent on the effector cell to target cell ratio. Using JTB18 NK cells and K562 targets, the release of proteoglycan was as high as 50% at an effector:target ratio of 0.5, and declined when the ratio was >1. When human NK cells were exposed to nonsusceptible target cells, only approximately 3% of their proteoglycans were exocytosed. Using six different clones of NK cells and seven target cell lines with differing susceptibilities to lysis, it was shown in another study (SCHMIDT et al. 1985) that the percentage release of proteoglycan from human NK cells was proportional to the ability of the NK cell to kill the tumor target. While direct contact with susceptible tumor cells results in exocytosis of proteoglycan from the NK cell, incubation of human NK cells with anti-T11 monoclonal antibodies will also result in the release of proteoglycans (SCHMIDT et al. 1988).

4.2 Interaction of Natural Killer Cell Serine Proteases with Proteoglycans

As discussed in detail elsewhere in this book, serine proteases with tryptic-like specificity may play a central role in cell-mediated killing because protease inhibitors such as DFP and phenylmethylsulfonylfluoride diminish the ability of mouse, rat, and human NK cells and cytotoxic thymus-dependent lymphocyte (CTL) to kill target cells. As is found in mast cells, these enzymes appear to be stored in the effector cell's secretory granules in an active state rather than as zymogens (PASTERNAK and EISEN 1985). The cDNAs that encode two different serine proteases have been isolated from mouse CTL-derived cDNA libraries (GERSHENFELD and WEISSMAN 1986; LOBE et al. 1986). The deduced amino acid sequence of one of these proteases revealed substantial homology with the MMC-derived enzyme RMCP-II. Considering the frequency of basic amino acids in both of these mouse CTL serine proteases, the enzymes would be expected to have strongly basic pIs. For example, the amino acid sequence derived from the cDNA of the mouse CTL protease described by LOBE et al. (1986) has 42 basic amino acids and only 12 acidic ones. In the one instance in which it has been determined, the pI of a serine protease present in a mouse CTL was found to be strongly basic (YOUNG et al. 1986).

Because NK cells and mast cells exhibit striking homology in their acidically charged, protease-resistant proteoglycans and in their basically charged serine proteases that are active at neutral pH, we suggested that one of the functions of proteoglycans in NK cells is to bind proteases. We have examined this in detail using human NK cells. Human cloned JT3 and JTB18 NK cells were radiolabeled with [^{35}S]sulfate and disrupted by nitrogen cavitation as described by MILLARD and coworkers (1984) for rat LGL tumor cells. After filtration through 5-µm and 3-µm filters, the liberated ^{35}S-labeled secretory granules were enriched by Percoll density gradient centrifugation. N-Benzyloxycarbonyl-L-lysine thiobenzyl ester (BLTe) was used as a substrate to detect the presence of tryptic-like enzymes. Similar to rodent CTL, human NK cells contain an enzyme that degrades BLTe in their secretory granules (M.M. KAMADA, J. MICHON, J. RITZ, W.E. SERAFIN, K.F. AUSTEN, R.P. MACDERMOTT, and R.L. STEVENS, unpublished data). This enzymatic activity has an optimum pH of 8.5. When ^{35}S-labeled human NK cell granules were disrupted by sonication and filtered on a column of Sepharose CL-2B equilibrated in phosphate buffered saline, the BLTe esterases filtered as a macromolecular complex along with approximately 8% of the cell's total ^{35}S-labeled proteoglycans (Fig. 4A). Treatment of the lysates with 4 M urea or nonionic detergents failed to dissociate the macromolecular complex, whereas the complex was dissociated in the presence of 3 M NaCl (Fig. 4B). Thus, like in mast cells, it appears that one of the functions of proteoglycans in NK cells is to bind serine proteases/esterases ionically to form large molecular weight complexes.

Because angiotensin I is susceptible to a variety of endopeptidases and exopeptidases (KLICKSTEIN and WINTROUB 1982; SERAFIN et al. 1987), isolated human NK cell granules were examined for proteases that would degrade this peptide. As assessed by high performance liquid chromatographic resolution of the digests, two peptides were generated which have retention times identical to des-Leu angiotensin I and angiotensin II. Amino acid analysis confirmed the identification of these two unknown peptides, indicating that human NK cells have a carboxypeptidase in their secretory granules. This carboxypeptidase-like exopeptidase has a pH optimum of 7.0 and therefore is clearly distinct from the BLTe esterase. Since the presence of exopeptidases in the secretory granules of NK cells and CTL has not been described, it remains to be seen whether this carboxypeptidase is one of the major proteins stored in the secretory granules of these effector cells. However, the presence in the secretory granules

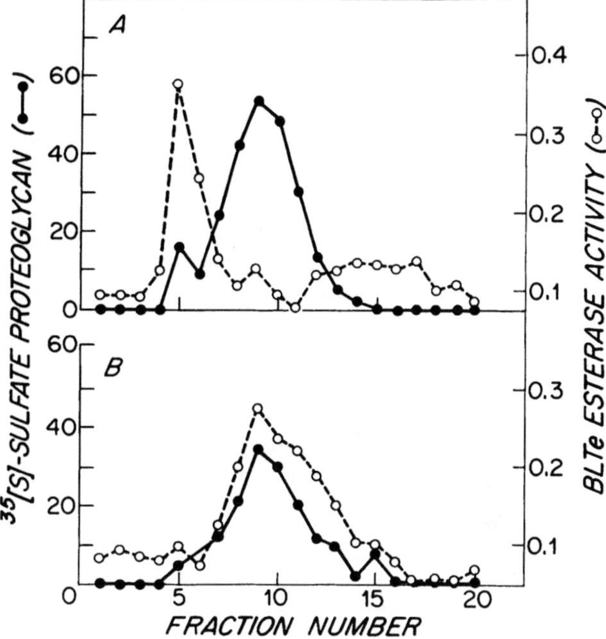

Fig. 4A, B. Sepharose CL-2B chromatography of human NK cell secretory granule-localized, ^{35}S-labeled proteoglycans (*solid circles*) and serine proteases/esterases that degrade BLTe (*open circles*). A The column was equilibrated and eluted with phosphate buffered saline. B The column was equilibrated and eluted with 3 *M* NaCl in phosphate buffered saline

of human NK cells of endopeptidases and exopeptidases packaged together with proteoglycans is reminiscent of what occurs in mast cells. This finding raises the possibility that these various enzymes participate in the coordinate degradation of common proteins.

References

Avraham S, Stevens RL, Gartner MC, Austen KF, Lalley PA, Weis JH (1988) Isolation of a cDNA that encodes the peptide core of the secretory granule proteoglycan of rat basophilic leukemia-1 cells and assessment of its homology to the human analogue. J Biol Chem 263:7292–7296

Benditt EP, Arase M, Roepper ME (1956) Histamine and heparin in isolated rat mast cells. J Histochem Cytochem 4:419–420

Benfey PN, Yin FH, Leder P (1987) Cloning of the mast cell protease, RMCP II. Evidence for cell-specific expression and a multi-gene family. J Biol Chem 262:5377–5384

Bland CE, Ginsburg H, Silbert JE, Metcalfe DD (1982) Mouse heparin proteoglycan. Synthesis by mast cell-fibroblast monolayers during lymphocyte-dependent mast cell proliferation. J Biol Chem 257:8661–8666

Bourdon MA, Oldberg A, Pierschbacher M, Ruoslahti E (1985) Molecular cloning and sequence analysis of a chondroitin sulfate proteoglycan cDNA. Proc Natl Acad Sci USA 82:1321–1325

Bourdon MA, Shiga M, Ruoslahti E (1986) Identification from cDNA of the precursor form of a chondroitin sulfate proteoglycan core protein. J Biol Chem 261:12534–12537

Bourdon MA, Krusius T, Campbell S, Schwartz NB, Ruoslahti E (1987a) Identification and synthesis of a recognition signal for the attachment of glycosaminoglycans to proteins. Proc Natl Acad Sci USA 84:3194–3198

Bourdon MA, Shiga M, Ruoslahti E (1987b) Gene expression of the chondroitin sulfate proteoglycan core protein PG19. Mol Cell Biol 7:33–40

Caulfield JP, Hein A, Tsunoda K, Shapiro R (1986) Detection of sulfur in fixed and embedded rat peritoneal mast cell granules by X-ray energy dispersive spectroscopy. J Electron Micro Tech 3:347–356

Claesson L, Larhammar D, Rask L, Petserson PA (1983) cDNA clone for the human invariant gamma chain of class II histocompatibility antigens and its implications for the protein structure. Proc Natl Acad Sci USA 80:7395–7399

DuBuske L, Austen KF, Czop J, Stevens RL (1984) Granule-associated serine neutral proteases of the mouse bone marrow-derived mast cell that degrade fibronectin: their increase after sodium butyrate treatment of the cells. J Immunol 133:1535–1541

Dvorak AM, Galli SJ, Marcum JA, Nabel G, der Simonian H, Goldin J, Monahan RA, Pyne K, Cantor H, Rosenberg RD, Dvorak HF (1983) Cloned mouse cells with natural killer function and cloned suppressor T cells express ultrastructural and biochemical features not shared by cloned inducer T cells. J Exp Med 157:843–861

Ehrlich P (1878) Beiträge zur Theorie und Praxis der Histologischen Färbung. Doctoral thesis, University of Leipzig, East Germany

Enerbäck L (1966) Mast cells in rat gastrointestinal mucosa. 2. Dye-binding and metachromatic properties. Acta Pathol Microbiol Scand 66:303–312

Everitt MT, Neurath H (1980) Rat peritoneal mast cell carboxypeptidase: localization, purification, and enzymatic properties. FEBS Lett 110:292–296

Gershenfeld HK, Weissman IL (1986) Cloning of a cDNA for a T cell-specific serine protease from a cytotoxic T lymphocyte. Science 232:854–857

Giacoletto KS, Sant AJ, Bono C, Gorka J, O'Sullivan DM, Quaranta V, Schwartz BD (1986) The human invariant chain is the core protein of the human class II-associated proteoglycan. J Exp Med 164:1422–1439

Horner AA (1971) Macromolecular heparin from rat skin. Isolation, characterization, and depolymerization with ascorbate. J Biol Chem 246:231–239

Isemura M, Ikenaka T (1975) β-Elimination and sulfite addition reaction of chondroitin sulfate peptidoglycan and the peptide structure of the linkage region. Biochim Biophys Acta 411:11–21

Klickstein LB, Wintroub BU (1982) Separation of angiotensins and assay of angiotensin-generating enzymes by high-performance liquid chromatography. Ann Biochem 120:146–150

Kolset SO, Seljelid R, Lindahl U (1984) Modulation of the morphology and glycosaminoglycan biosynthesis of human monocytes, induced by culture substrates. Biochem J 219:793–799

Krusius T, Ruoslahti E (1986) Primary structure of an extracellular matrix proteoglycan core protein deduced from cloned cDNA. Proc Natl Acad Sci USA 83:7683–7687

Lagunoff D, Pritzl P (1976) Characterization of rat mast cell granule proteins. Arch Biochem Biophys 173:554–563

Levitt D, Ho PL (1983) Induction of chondroitin sulfate proteoglycan synthesis and secretion in lymphocytes and monocytes. J Cell Biol 97:351–358

Lindahl U, Cifonelli JA, Lindahl B, Rodén L (1965) The role of serine in the linkage of heparin to protein. J Biol Chem 240:2817–2820

Lobe CG, Finlay BP, Paranchych W, Paetkau VH, Bleackley RC (1986) Novel serine proteases encoded by two cytotoxic T lymphocyte-specific genes. Science 232:858–861

Luikart SD, Maniglia CA, Sartorelli AC (1984) Glycosaminoglycan synthesis during differentiation of HL60/HGPRT$^-$ leukemia cells induced by dimethyl sulfoxide and 12-O-tetradecanoylphorbol-13-acetate. Cancer Res 44:2907–2912

MacDermott RP, Schmidt RE, Caulfield JP, Hein A, Bartley GT, Ritz J, Schlossman SF, Austen KF, Stevens RL (1985) Proteoglycans in cell-mediated cytotoxicity. Identification, localization, and exocytosis of a chondroitin sulfate proteoglycan from human cloned natural killer cells during target cell lysis. J Exp Med 162:1771–1787

Metcalfe DD, Lewis RA, Silbert JE, Rosenberg RD, Wasserman SI, Austen KF (1979) Isolation and characterization of heparin from human lung. J Clin Invest 64:1537–1543

Metcalfe DD, Smith JA, Austen KF, Silbert JE (1980a) Polydispersity of rat mast cell heparin. J Biol Chem 255:11753–11758

Metcalfe DD, Wasserman SI, Austen KF (1980b) Isolation and characterization of sulphated mucopolysaccharides from rat leukaemic (RBL-1) basophils. Biochem J 185:367–372

Metcalfe DD, Litvin J, Wasserman SI (1982) The isolation, identification and characterization of sulfated glycosaminoglycans synthesized in vitro by human eosinophils. Biochim Biophys Acta 715:196–204

Millard PJ, Henkart MP, Reynolds CW, Henkart PA (1984) Purification and properties of cytoplasmic granules from cytotoxic rat LGL tumors. J Immunol 132:3197–3204

Muir H (1958) The nature of the link between protein and carbohydrate of a chondroitin sulphate complex from hyaline cartilage. Biochem J 69:195–204

Ogren S, Lindahl U (1975) Cleavage of macromolecular heparin by an enzyme from mouse mastocytoma. J Biol Chem 250:2690–2697

Ohhashi Y, Hasumi F, Mori Y (1984) Comparative study on glycosaminoglycans synthesized in peripheral and peritoneal polymorphonuclear leucocytes from guinea pigs. Biochem J 217:199–207

Oldberg A, Hayman EG, Ruoslahti E (1981) Isolation of a chondroitin sulfate proteoglycan from a rat yolk sac tumor and immunochemical demonstration of its cell surface location. J Biol Chem 256:10847–10852

Oldberg A, Antonsson P, Heinegård D (1987) The partial amino acid sequence of bovine cartilage proteoglycan, deduced from a cDNA clone, contains numerous Ser-Gly sequences arranged in homologous repeats. Biochem J 243:255–259

Olsson I (1969) Intracellular distribution and sites of synthesis of glycosaminoglycans (mucopolysaccharides) in human leukocytes. Exp Cell Res 54:314–317

Orenstein NS, Galli SJ, Dvorak AM, Silbert JE, Dvorak HF (1978) Sulfated glycosaminoglycans of guinea pig basophilic leukocytes. J Immunol 121:586–592

Parmley RT, Rahemtulla F, Cooper MD, Rodén L (1985) Ultrastructural and biochemical characterization of glycosaminoglycans in HNK-1-positive large granular lymphocytes. Blood 66:20–25

Pasternak MS, Eisen HN (1985) A novel serine esterase expressed by cytotoxic T lymphocytes. Nature 314:743–745

Razin E, Stevens RL, Akiyama F, Schmid K, Austen KF (1982) Culture from mouse bone marrow of a subclass of mast cells possessing a distinct chondroitin sulfate proteoglycan with glycosaminoglycans rich in N-acetylgalactosamine-4,6-disulfate. J Biol Chem 257:7229–7236

Reynolds CW, Bere EW, Ward JM (1984) Natural killer activity in the rat. III. Characterization of transplantable large granular lymphocyte (LGL) leukemias in the F344 rat. J Immunol 132:534–540

Robinson HC, Horner AA, Höök M, Ogren S, Lindahl U (1978) A proteoglycan form of heparin and its degradation to single-chain molecules. J Biol Chem 253:6687–6693

Rodén L (1980) Structure and metabolism of connective tissue proteoglycans. In: Lennarz WJ (ed) The biochemistry of glycoproteins and proteoglycans. Plenum, New York, pp 267–371

Rothenberg ME, Caulfield JP, Austen KF, Hein A, Edmiston K, Newburger PE, Stevens RL (1987) Biochemical and morphological characterization of basophilic leukocytes from two patients with myelogenous leukemia. J Immunol 138:2616–2625

Sage H, Woodbury RG, Bornstein P (1979) Structural studies on human type IV collagen. J Biol Chem 254:9893–9900

Schmidt RE, MacDermott RP, Bartley G, Bertovich M, Amato DA, Austen KF, Schlossman SF, Stevens RL, Ritz J (1985) Specific release of proteoglycans from human natural killer cells during target cell lysis. Nature 318:289–291

Schmidt RE, Caulfield JP, Michon J, Hein A, Kamada MM, MacDermott RP, Stevens RL, Ritz J (1988) T11/CD2 activation of cloned human natural killer cells results in increased conjugate formation and exocytosis of cytolytic granules. J Immunol 140:991–1002

Schwartz LB, Bradford TR (1986) Regulation of tryptase from human lung mast cells by heparin. Stabilization of the active tetramer. J Biol Chem 261:7372–7379

Schwartz LB, Riedel C, Caulfield JP, Wasserman SI, Austen KF (1981) Cell association of complexes of chymase, heparin proteoglycan, and protein after degranulation by rat mast cells. J Immunol 126:2071–2078

Seldin DC, Seno N, Austen KF, Stevens RL (1984) Analysis of polysulfated chondroitin disaccharides by high-performance liquid chromatography. Ann Biochem 141:291–300

Seldin DC, Austen KF, Stevens RL (1985) Purification and characterization of protease-resistant secretory granule proteoglycans containing chondroitin sulfate di-B and heparin-like glycosaminoglycans from rat basophilic leukemia cells. J Biol Chem 260:11131–11139

Serafin WE, Katz HR, Austen KF, Stevens RL (1986) Complexes of heparin proteoglycans, chondroitin sulfate E proteoglycans, and [^{3}H]diisopropyl fluorophosphate-binding proteins are exocytosed from activated mouse bone marrow-derived mast cells. J Biol Chem 261:15017–15021

Serafin WE, Dayton ET, Gravallese PM, Austen KF, Stevens RL (1987) Carboxypeptidase A in mouse mast cells. Identification, characterization, and use as a differentiation marker. J Immunol 139:3771–3776

Smith TJ, Hougland MW, Johnson DA (1984) Human lung tryptase. Purification and characterization. J Biol Chem 259:11046–11051

Stevens RL, Otsu K, Austen KF (1985) Purification and analysis of the core protein of the protease-resistant intracellular chondroitin sulfate E proteoglycan from the interleukin 3-dependent mouse mast cell. J Biol Chem 260:14194–14200

Stevens RL, Lee TDG, Seldin DC, Austen KF, Befus AD, Bienenstock J (1986) Intestinal mucosal mast cells from rats infected with Nippostrongylus brasiliensis contain protease-resistant chondroitin sulfate di-B proteoglycans. J Immunol 137:291–295

Stevens RL, Otsu K, Weis JH, Tantravahi RV, Austen KF, Henkart PA, Galli MC, Reynolds CW (1987) Co-sedimentation of chondroitin sulfate A glycosaminoglycans and proteoglycans with the cytolytic secretory granules of rat large granular lymphocyte (LGL) tumor cells, and identification of a mRNA in normal and transformed LGL that encodes proteoglycans. J Immunol 139:863–868

Stevens RL, Fox CC, Lichtenstein LM, Austen KF (1988a) Identification of chondroitin sulfate E proteoglycans and heparin proteoglycans in the secretory granules of human lung mast cells. Proc Natl Acad Sci USA 85:2284–2287

Stevens RL, Avraham S, Gartner MC, Bruns GAP, Austen KF, Weis JH (1988b) Isolation and characterization of a cDNA that encodes the peptide core of the secretory granule proteoglycan of human promyelocytic leukemia HL-60 cells. J Biol Chem 263:7287–7291

Tantravahi RV, Stevens RL, Austen KF, Weis JH (1986) A single gene in mast cells encodes the core peptides of heparin and chondroitin sulfate proteoglycans. Proc Natl Acad Sci USA 83:9207–9210

Trong HL, Neurath H, Woodbury RG (1987) Substrate specificity of the chymotrypsin-like protease in secretory granules isolated from rat mast cells. Proc Natl Acad Sci USA 84:364–367

Vartio T, Seppä H, Vaheri A (1981) Susceptibility of soluble and matrix fibronectins to degradation by tissue proteinases, mast cell chymase and cathepsin G. J Biol Chem 256:471–477

Woodbury RG, Neurath H (1978) Purification of an atypical mast cell protease and its levels in developing rats. Biochemistry 17:4298–4304

Young JD, Leong LG, Liu CC, Damiano A, Wall DA, Cohn ZA (1986) Isolation and characterization of a serine esterase from cytolytic T cell granules. Cell 47:183–194

Yurt RW, Leid RW, Austen KF, Silbert JE (1977a) Native heparin from rat peritoneal mast cells. J Biol Chem 252:518–521

Yurt RW, Leid RW, Spragg J, Austen KF (1977b) Immunologic release of heparin from purified rat peritoneal mast cells. J Immunol 118:1201–1207

Yurt R, Austen KF (1977c) Preparative purification of the rat mast cell chymase. Characterization and interaction with granule components. J Exp Med 146:1405–1419

The Homologous Species Restriction of the Complement Attack: Structure and Function of the C8 Binding Protein

G.M. Hänsch

1 Introduction   109
2 Identification of the C8bp   109
3 Functional Characterization of C8bp   111
4 Mode of Inhibition   112
5 Comparison of C8bp with Other Complement or Complement Regulatory Protein   113
6 Presence of C8bp in Nucleated Cells   114
7 Lack of C8bp in Leukocytes and Platelets of PNH-Patients   115
8 Biological Relevance of C8bp   116
9 Conclusion   117
References   117

1 Introduction

The homologous restriction of the complement attack, i.e., the inability of complement to lyse erythrocytes of the same species, has long been known (BORDET 1900), but only in the last decade has progress been made in understanding the nature of this phenomenon. It has become evident that the complement sequence is inhibited species-specifically on the membrane at two steps at least (SHIN et al. 1986), thus protecting the erythrocytes against the complement attack. Inhibition is accomplished by two membrane proteins: one, the so-called decay accelerating factor (DAF) which inhibits the complement activation phase (NICHOLSON-WELLER et al. 1982), and the other, the C8 binding protein (C8bp) which interferes with the action of the late complement components (SCHÖNER-MARK et al. 1984, 1986). Since the late complement components C5b-9 represent the cytolytic effector phase of complement, the following discussion will be restricted to the function and characterization of the C8bp.

2 Identification of the C8bp

Studying the late complement components' lysis of various erythrocytes, it was learned that the extent of lysis varies greatly with the species of C8 and C9 if the erythrocyte carries only a limited number of C5b-7 sites (LACHMANN

Institut für Immunologie der Universität Heidelberg, Heidelberg, Federal Republic of Germany

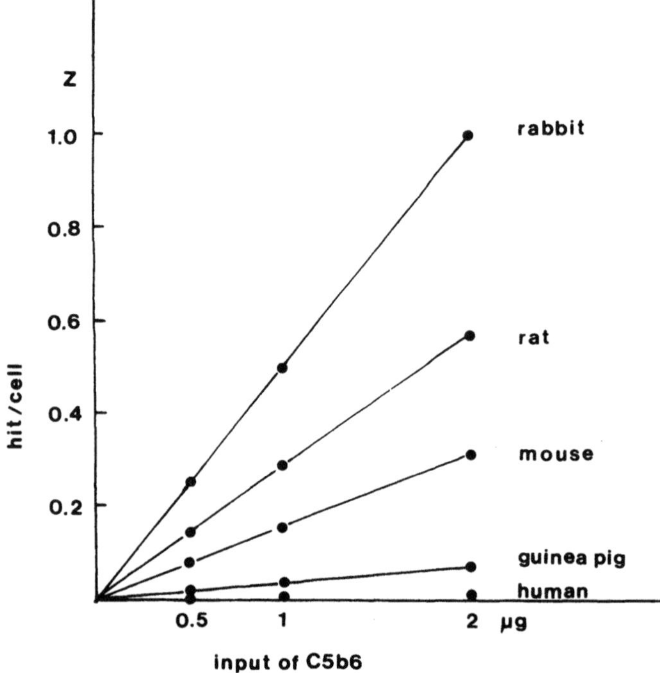

Fig. 1. Species-specific dependency of the degree of lysis for C8 and C9: human erythrocytes carrying limited amounts of C5b67 as determined by the input of preactivated C5b6 (*abscissa*) were lyzed with an excess of C8 and C9 from various species. The lytic efficiency was calculated as hit/cell (*ordinate*)

et al. 1973; YAMAMOTO 1977; HÄNSCH et al. 1981) (Fig. 1). In all erythrocyte species, however, lysis was least efficient when C8 and C9 were from the same species as the target erythrocyte, a phenomenon which we termed "homologous species restriction" (HÄNSCH et al. 1981). For the lysis of human erythrocyte the species of C8 was important, e.g., rabbit C8 together with rabbit or human C9 was efficient in lysing human erythrocytes carrying human C5b-7, whereas human C8 was not (SCHÖNERMARK et al. 1986). Binding of C8, however, was not inhibited, pointing to the possibility that lysis was inhibited at the C8–C9 step, and moreover, that C8 was recognized as "self" on the membrane. In subsequent studies a membrane protein with affinity for C8 was identified in the erythrocyte membrane (SCHÖNERMARK et al. 1986) (Fig. 2). It is a glycoprotein with a molecular weight of 65 KD, as estimated by sodium dodecyl sulfate-polyacrylamide gel electrophoresis (SDS-PAGE). Called C8 binding protein (C8bp) because of its affinity for C8, it is apparently deeply embedded in the membrane as it is resistant to stripping by proteolytic enzymes. C8bp, however, can be removed by a phosphatidylinositol-specific phospholipase C (PIPLC) (PI) indicating that C8bp is anchored to the membrane via phosphatidylinositol (HÄNSCH et al. 1988), similar to DAF, acetylcholine esterase, and to lymphocyte antigens (DAVITZ et al. 1986; LOW and FINEAN 1977).

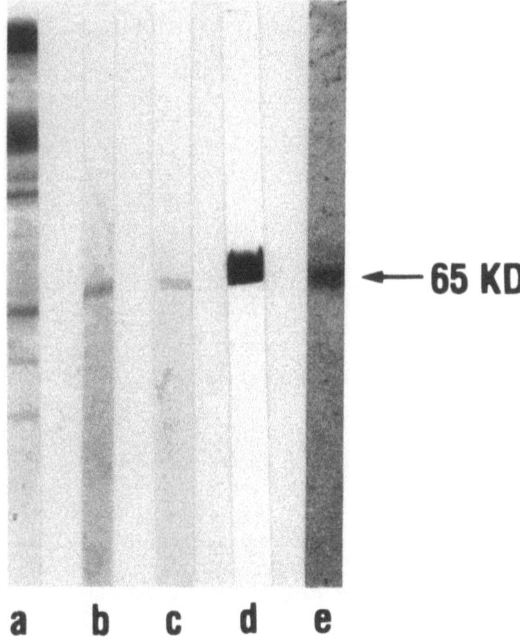

Fig. 2a–e. The C8 binding protein of the erythrocyte membrane: Erythrocytes were osmolysed, separated by SDS-PAGE (**a**) and blotted. Isolated C8 was added to the blot, and binding of C8 was tested with anti-C8 (lane **b**). With an antibody raised against purified C8bp a major band was seen in the area of 65 KD (**c**). Lane **d** shows the isolated C8bp with SDS-PAGE separation (silver stain) and immunoblot (**e**)

3 Functional Characterization of C8bp

For functional analysis, C8bp was isolated from the membranes. Since C8bp was resistant to papain stripping, papain-treated erythrocytes were osmolyzed and membrane proteins were extracted by phenol-water. Approximately 35 mg lyophilized protein were obtained from 12 l of blood, and from this crude protein extract C8bp was purified, either by isoelectric focusing, or by gel filtration. This yield has an average of 1–5 mg C8bp homogenous, as judged by SDS-PAGE analysis (Fig. 2). The isolated C8bp retained its functional activity in that it inhibits the lysis of erythrocytes, e.g., chicken or guinea pig erythrocytes by human C5b-9. Lysis was inhibited at the C8 stage, but only when C8 was of human origin. Taken together, the data suggest that C8bp is the membrane constituent responsible for the homologous restriction.

Studies on erythrocytes from patients suffering from paroxysmal nocturnal hemoglobinuria (PNH) type III supported this hypothesis: erythrocytes of PNH type III differ from normal E as they are sensitive to lysis by human C5b-9 (Rosse 1973; Packman et al. 1979); thus the homologous species restriction is obviously lost (for review see Rosse 1986). Indeed, PNH type III lack C8bp in addition to lacking DAF and acetylcholinesterase (AChE). Isolated C8bp, when reincorporated into the PNH-E, restored the species restriction (Hänsch et al. 1987). Interestingly enough, just 1000 molecules/E are sufficient to inhibit the lysis (Fig. 3).

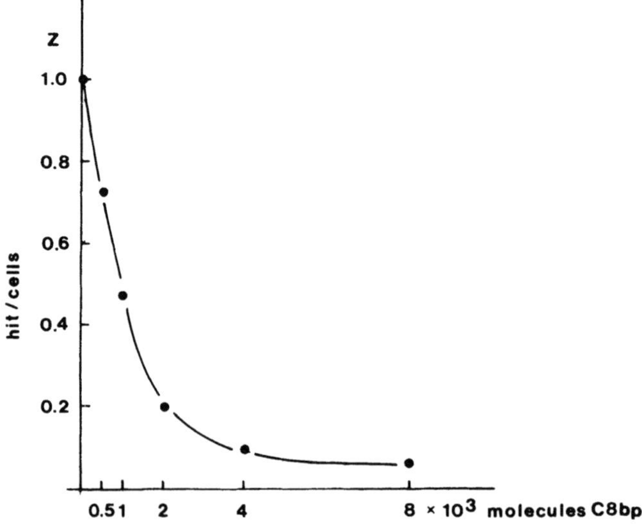

Fig. 3. Inhibition of C5b-9-mediated PNH-E lysis by C8bp: [^{125}I] C8bp was incorporated into PNH-E. Uptake was quantitated by measuring radioactivity associated with membranes (*abscissa*). The E were then lysed with C5b-9, and the extent of lysis was calculated as hit/cell (*ordinate*)

4 Mode of Inhibition

How C8bp inhibits lysis is not yet understood. Binding of C5b-8 to the homologous E is not inhibited, congruent with the fact that binding of C8 to C5b-7 is mediated by the C8 β-chain, whereas C8bp interacts with the C8α–γ subunit. Moreover, binding of C5b-7 and of C8 to PNH-E type III (=C8bp deficient E) is also not enhanced (ROSENFELD et al. 1985; HU and NICHOLSON-WELLER 1985). Thus, C8bp most probably interferes with a postbinding event, i.e., interaction of C8 with C9, and/or insertion of the C5b-9 into the bilayer, two reactions which are mediated by the C8 α-chain. Indeed, insertion efficiency is decreased in the homologous system (HU and SHIN 1984), whereas enhanced C9 uptake is seen in C8bp-deficient PNH type III cells (HU and NICHOLSON-WELLER 1985), as well as a greater degree of lysis per C9 molecule bound (PARKER et al. 1985). Studying C8bp-reconstituted erythrocytes, C8bp was found within the C5b-9 complex when E (e.g., sheep) were loaded with radiolabeled C8bp and lysed by human complement (Fig. 4) (SCHÖNERMARK et al. 1988).

As an indicator of C8–C9 interaction, C5b-8-dependent polymerization of C9 was studied in the presence and absence of C8bp, since induction of C9 polymerization is probably mediated by the C8α-chain (TSCHOPP et al. 1985). It was found that C8bp inhibited C9 polymerization in erythrocytes (e.g., sheep) lysed by large amounts of human complement (SCHÖNERMARK et al. 1987). Support for these data was derived again from studies of PNH-E erythrocytes. In contrast to normal human E, PNH-E show an extensive C9 polymerization (HU and NICHOLSON-WELLER 1985), which can be inhibited by isolated C8bp (HÄNSCH et al. 1987) (Fig. 5).

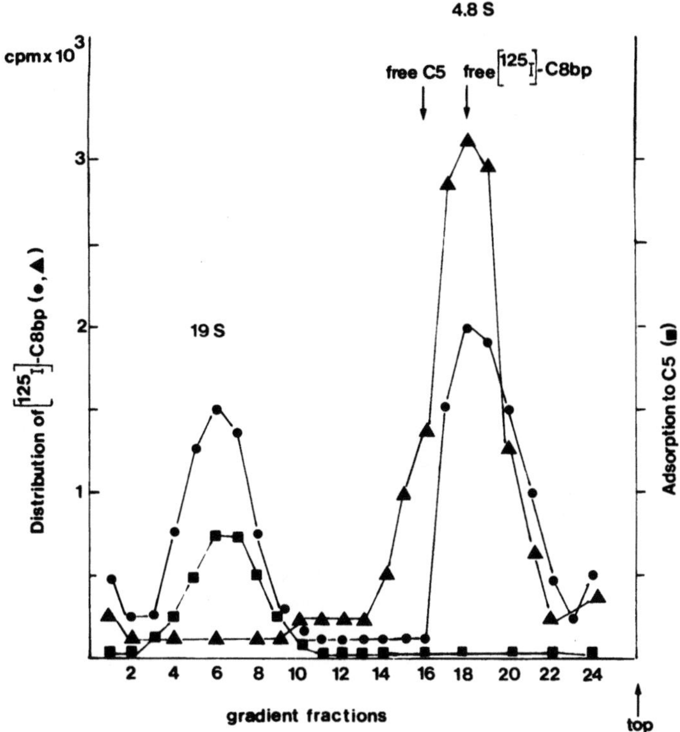

Fig. 4. Density gradient centrifugation of complement-lysed sheep-erythrocyte (E) membranes having incorporated [125I] C8bp: [125I] C8bp was added to sheep E. The E were either lysed by antibody and complement (*circles*) or by buffer in low ionic strength (*triangles*). After extraction of the membrane proteins with detergent, in the case of the complement-lysed E the radioactivity was found in two peaks of approximately 19S and 4.8S (*circles*); after osmolysis only the 4.8S peak was seen (*triangles*), corresponding to the sedimentation rate of isolated C8bp. The radioactivity of the 19S peak could be adsorbed to anti-C5 (*squares*), whereas the 4.8S could not

5 Comparison of C8bp with Other Complement or Complement Regulatory Proteins

Because of its function as a regulatory protein of the complement sequence, and also because of other properties (size, PI anchoring, deficiency in PNH), a similarity of C8bp to DAF was sought. C8bp, however, has no effect on the stability of C3-convertase (SCHÖNERMARK et al. 1986) and, furthermore, anti-DAF which abolishes down-regulation of the C3-convertase did not affect the species restriction of the late complement proteins (SHIN et al. 1986). C8bp is also antigenetically different from AChE, even though they share two properties: PI anchor and lack in PNH.

Furthermore, a relationship of C8bp to the S-protein was tested because they share at least one functional property: inhibition of C9 polymerization (PODACK et al. 1984). However, antibodies to S-protein did not react with purified C8bp nor with any other erythrocyte membrane protein.

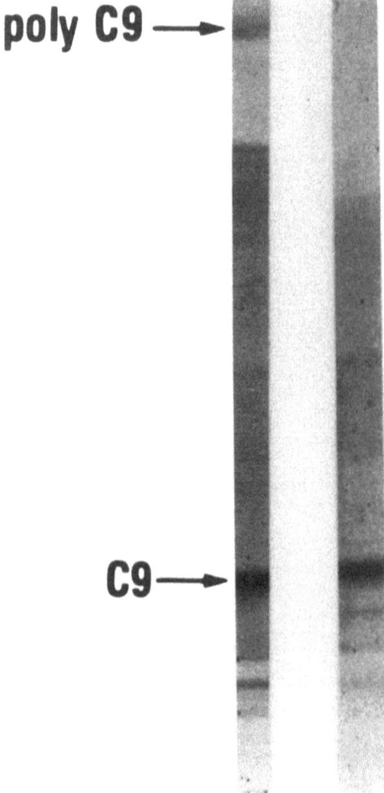

Fig. 5. Inhibition of C9 polymerization by C8bp: Erythrocytes (C sheep E) show C9 polymerization when lysed by antibody and human complement. When C8bp was incorporated into the membranes, C9 polymerization was inhibited

More surprising was the fact that antibodies to C8 and to C9 also reacted with C8bp and vice versa; specifically, anti-C8bp recognized the C8α-chain. These data suggest a partial homology between C8bp, C8α-chain, and C9. Further confirmation derives from affinity studies in which C8bp not only showed a high affinity for the whole C8 molecule, but also for the isolated C8γ-chain, thus behaving similarly to C8α (SCHÖNERMARK et al. 1988).

Independent of this description of C8bp, another membrane protein, the so-called homologous restriction factor (HRF), was described. HRF was purified according to its affinity for C8 and C9 and was described as a 32- and 65-KD membrane protein (ZALMAN et al. 1986). HRF is deficient in PNH-patients and shares many functional and biochemical properties with C8bp (ZALMAN et al. 1987). Therefore, there is a good possibility that HRF is identical to C8bp.

6 Presence of C8bp in Nucleated Cells

Using polyclonal antibodies to C8bp, leukocytes and leukocyte cell lines were screened for the presence of C8bp. C8bp was found in the leukocytes and

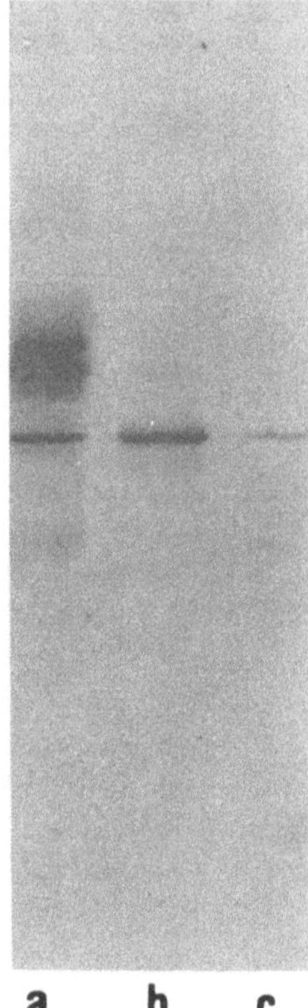

Fig. 6a–c. Demonstration of C8bp in the membranes of nucleated cells: after separation by SDS-PAGE of membranes of **a** monocytes, **b** polymorphonuclear leukocytes, or **c** platelets in the immunoblot with anti-C8bp, a band was seen in the area of 50 KD

in several cell lines (e.g., HL-60, Raji, K 562). It is of interest to note that the protein recognized by the anti-C8bp (Fig. 6) was slightly smaller than the erythrocyte-derived C8bp (C8bpE). The isolated 50 KD protein (e.g., purified from thrombocytes, C8bpT) had functional activities similar to the C8bpE, i.e., it inhibited the C5b-9-mediated lysis of E (BLAAS et al. 1988).

7 Lack of C8bp in Leukocytes and Platelets of PNH-Patients

To study the function of C8bp in the membrane of cells other than erythrocytes, resort was again made to cells of PNH-patients. Leukocytes and platelets of PNH patients lacked C8bp (Fig. 6) (BLAAS et al. 1988). Thus, in addition to the DAF-deficiency, platelets also showed a second membrane protein defect. Platelets of PNH-patients, however, have a normal lifetime in vivo (DEVINE et al. 1987), suggesting that they are not lysed by complement.

Besides lysis, sublytic concentrations of C5b-9 also stimulate various cell functions (IMAGAWA et al. 1983; BETZ and HÄNSCH 1984; HÄNSCH et al. 1984). More specifically, platelets respond to C5b-9 with an enhanced thromboxane

Table 1. Release of thromboxane TXB_2 and serotonin from platelets of PNH patients by C5b-9

Platelets incubated with C5b-9[a]	TXB_2 (ng/ml)	Serotonin (% specific release)
Patient I	10.2	26
+C8bp (0.5 µg)	1.5	0
Patient II	28.2	40.8
+C8bp (0.5 µg)	7.4	12.0
Healthy		
Control I	2.2	0
Control II	2.4	0

[a] 0.1 ml platelets (10^8) were incubated with purified C5b6 (10 µg), C7 (20 µg), C8 (5 µg) and C9 (10 µg) added consecutively for 60 min at 37° C

synthesis (POLLEY et al. 1981; HÄNSCH et al. 1985; BETZ et al. 1987). In platelets of PNH patients, the thromboxane and serotonin release in response to C5b-9 was dramatically enhanced, compared with what occurs in platelets of normal donors. Isolated C8bp (E- or platelet-derived) inhibited the C5b-9-mediated release, suggesting that lack of C8bp might not only enhance the lytic activity of C5b-9 but also its stimulatory activity (data shown for two patients in Table 1) (BLAAS et al. 1988).

8 Biological Relevance of C8bp

The question of whether or not a biological structure is of any advantage for the individual or the species is always difficult to answer, but it is also very intriguing. In the case of C8bp, the question is why should there be another regulatory protein for the late components when the complement sequence is already down-regulated at the C3-level? After studying the action of the late components it became obvious that C5b-9, once activated, can bind to virtually all membranes without discriminating between the activating particle (e.g., antibody-coated bacteria, immune complexes) and the body's own tissue. Even though the lifetime of the C5b-9 is limited due to loss of the membrane binding site during fluid-phase complex formation (LACHMANN and THOMPSON 1970; GÖTZE and MÜLLER-EBERHARD 1970) and due to fluid-phase regulatory protein, e.g., S-protein (PODACK et al. 1977) or lipoprotein (LINT et al. 1977; PODACK et al. 1978), cells in the immediate vicinity of the site of complement activation are targets for C5b-9 ("innocent bystander lysis", GÖTZE and MÜLLER-EBERHARD 1970). Indeed, C5b-9, which is activated on the surface of complement-resistant bacteria, can be transferred in a lytically active form to erythrocytes ("deviated lysis"; ROTHER et al. 1974).

Normal human E are resistant to lysis by C5b-9; however, when C8bp is missing, as in the case of PNH type III, lysis will occur, leading eventually to anemia. How a C8bp defect affects the viability and function of nucleated cells is not yet clear. Platelets respond with an enhanced mediator release, e.g., thromboxane release, which could contribute to the thrombotic complications seen in some PNH patients.

9 Conclusion

Erythrocyte and leukocyte membranes contain the protein C8bp, which by binding C8 inhibits the C5b-9-mediated lysis as well as the C5b-9-induced mediator release in a species-specific manner.

The biological importance of a membrane protein protecting the cell against the attack by homologous complement is evident: It minimizes self-destruction without impairing the host defense.

References

Betz M, Hänsch GM (1984) Release of arachidonic acid: a new function of the late complement components. Immunobiology 166:473–483

Betz M, Seitz M, Hänsch GM (1987) Thromboxane B_2 synthesis in human platelets induced by the late complement components C5b-9. Int Arch Allergy Appl Immunol 82:313–316

Blaas P, Berger B, Weber S, Peter HH, Hänsch GM (1988) Paroxysmal nocturnal hemoglobinuria (PNH) type III: enhanced stimulation of platelets by the terminal complement components is related to the lack of C8bp in the membrane. J Immunol 140:3045–3051

Bordet J (1900) Les serums hemolytique, les antitoxines et les theories des serum cytolytiques. Ann Inst Pasteur 14:257–271

Davitz MA, Low MG, Nussenzweig V (1986) Release of decay-accelerating factor (DAF) from the cell membrane by phosphatidylinositol-specific phospholipase C. J Exp Med 163:1150–1161

Devine DV, Siegel RS, Rosse WF (1987) Interaction of the platelets in paroxysmal nocturnal hemoglobinuria with complement. J Clin Invest 79:131–137

Götze O, Müller-Eberhard HJ (1970) Lysis of erythrocytes by complement in the absence of antibody. J exp Med 132:898–903

Hänsch GM, Hammer C, Vanguri P, Shin ML (1981) Self versus nonself restriction in the lysis of erythrocytes by the terminal complement proteins. Proc Natl Acad Sci USA 78:5118–5122

Hänsch GM, Seitz M, Martinotti G, Betz M, Rauterberg EW, Gemsa D (1984) Macrophages release arachidonic acid, prostaglandin E_2 and thromboxane in response to the late complement components. J Immunol 133:2145–2150

Hänsch GM, Gemsa D, Resch K (1985) Induction of prostanoid synthesis in human platelets by the late complement components C5b-9 and channel forming antibiotic nystatin: inhibition of reacylation of liberated arachidonic acid. J Immunol 135:1320–1324

Hänsch GM, Schönermark S, Roelcke D (1987) Paroxysmal nocturnal hemoglobinuria type III: lack of an erythrocyte membrane protein restricting the lysis by C5b-9. J Clin Invest 80:7–12

Hänsch GM, Weller P, Nicholson-Weller A (1988) Release of C8bp from the cell membrane by phosphatidylinositol-specific phospholipase C. Blood (in press)

Hu V, Nicholson-Weller A (1985) Enhanced complement-mediated lysis of type III paroxysmal nocturnal hemoglobinuria erythrocytes involves increased C9 binding and polymerisation. Proc Natl Acad Sci USA 82:5520–5524

Hu V, Shin ML (1984) Species-restricted target cell lysis by human complement. Complement-lysed erythrocytes from different species differ in the ratio of bound and inserted C9. J Immunol 133:2133–2137

Imagawa DK, Osifchin NE, Paznekas WA, Shin ML, Mayer MM (1983) Consequences of cell membrane attack by complement: release of arachidonate and formation of inflammatory mediators. Proc Natl Acad Sci USA 80:6647–6651

Lachmann PJ, Thompson RA (1970) Reactive lysis: the complement-mediated lysis of unsensitized cells. II. The characterization of activated reactor as C5b6 and the participation of C8 and C9. J Exp Med 131:643–657

Lachmann PJ, Bowyer DE, Nicol P, Dawson RMC, Munn EA (1973) Studies on the terminal stages of complement lysis. Immunology 24:135–145

Lint TF, Behrends CL, Gewurz H (1977) Serum lipoproteins and C567-INH activity. J Immunol 119:883–888

Low MG, Finean JB (1977) Non-lytic release of acetylcholinesterase from erythrocytes by a phosphatidylinositol-specific phospholipase C. FEBS Lett 82:143–146

Nicholson-Weller A, Burger J, Fearon DT, Weller PF, Austen KF (1982) Isolation of human erythrocyte membrane glycoprotein with decay-accelerating activity for C3-convertases of the complement system. J Immunol 129:184–189

Packman CH, Rosenfeld SI, Jenkins DE, Thiem PA, Leddy JP (1979) Complement lysis of human erythrocytes. Differing susceptibility of two types of paroxysmal nocturnal hemoglobinuria cells to C5b-9. J Clin Invest 64:428–433

Parker CJ, Wiedmer T, Sims PJ, Rosse WF (1985) Characterization of the complement sensitivity of paroxysmal nocturnal hemoglobinuria erythrocytes. J Clin Invest 75:2074–2084

Podack ER, Kolb WP, Müller-Eberhard HJ (1977) The SC5b-7 complex: formation, isolation, properties and subunit composition. J Immunol 119:2024–2029

Podack ER, Kolb WP, Müller-Eberhard HJ (1978) The C5b6 complex: formation, isolation and inhibition of its activity by lipoprotein and the S-protein of human serum. J Immunol 120:1841–1848

Podack ER, Preissner KT, Müller-Eberhard HJ (1984) Inhibition of C9 polymerization within the SC5b-9 complex of complement by S-protein. Acta Pathol Microbiol Immunol Scand [Suppl] [C] 284:89–96

Polley MJ, Nachman RL, Weksler BB (1981) Human complement in the arachidonic acid transformation pathway in platelets. J Exp Med 153:257–268

Rosenfeld SI, Jenkins DE, Leddy JP (1985) Enhanced reactive lysis of paroxysmal nocturnal hemoglobinuria cells does not involve increased C7 binding or cell bound C3b. J Immunol 134:506–510

Rosse WF (1973) Variations in the complement-sensitive cells in paroxysmal nocturnal hemoglobinuria. Br J Haematol 24:327–342

Rosse WF (1986) The control of complement activation by the blood cells ion paroxysmal nocturnal hemoglobinuria. Blood 67:268–269

Rother U, Hänsch GM, Menzel J, Rother K (1974) Deviated lysis: transfer of complement lytic activity to unsensitized cells. Generation of a transferable activity on the surface of complement-resistent bacteria. Z Immunitaetsforsch 148:172–178

Schönermark S, Rauterberg EW, Roelcke D, Löke S, Hänsch GM (1984) A C8-binding protein on the surface of human erythrocytes: the inhibition of lysis in a homologous system (abstract). Immunobiology 168:109

Schönermark S, Rauterberg EW, Shin ML, Löke S, Roelcke D, Hänsch GM (1986) Homologous species restriction in lysis of human erythrocytes. A membrane-derived protein with C8-binding capacity functions as an inhibitor. J Immunol 136:1772–1776

Schönermark S, Filsinger S, Berger B, Hänsch GM (1988) The C8 binding protein of the human erythrocyte: interaction with the components of the complement attack phase. Immunology 63:585–590

Shin ML, Hänsch GM, Hu V, Nicholson-Weller A (1986) Membrane factor(s) responsible for homologous species restriction of complement-mediated lysis: evidence for a factor other than DAF operating at the stage of C8 and C9. Immunology 136:1777–1782

Tschopp J, Podack ER, Müller-Eberhard HJ (1985) The membrane attack complex of complement: C5b-8 complex as accelerator of C9 polymerization. J Immunol 134:495–499

Yamamoto K (1977) Lytic activity of C5-9 complexes for erythrocytes from species other than sheep: C9 rather than C8-dependent lytic activity. J Immunol 119:1482–1487

Zalman LS, Wood LM, Müller-Eberhard HJ (1986) Isolation of a human erythrocyte membrane protein capable of inhibiting expression of homologous complement channels. Proc Natl Acad Sci USA 83:6975–6979

Zalman LS, Wood LM, Frank MM, Müller-Eberhard HJ (1987) Deficiency of the homologous restriction factor in paroxysmal nocturnal hemoglobinuria. J Exp Med 165:572–577

Subject Index

acetylcholine esterase 110
activated cytotoxic T lymphocytes 81
activation, CTL 75
activity, cytolytic 69
–, transcriptional 75
affinity 36
Arg-Gly-Asp sequences 25

blot, Northern 39
–, Southern 39

Ca chelator, intracellular 5
carbohydrate 35
–, granzyme A 35
CCPI 70, 73, 82
–, cleavage specificities 82
–, human CTLs 83
–, Intron positions 73
–, serine protease cascade 83, 89–90
CCPII 73
–, Intron positions 73
cell lysis, complemented-mediated 19
chromatin-formation 75
cloning 38
complement 34
–, proteins, C5b 21
–, –, C5b-7 19
–, –, C5b-8 19, 54
–, –, C5b-9 19
–, –, C8 19, 21
–, –, –, amino acid sequences of human α sub-
    unit 23
–, –, –, binding protein (C8bp) 109
–, –, –, cDNA clones for α, β, γ 23
–, –, –, deficiencies, human 23
–, –, –, epidermal growth factor precursor
    (EGFP) 24
–, –, –, functional organization 20
–, –, –, α genes 23
–, –, –, β genes 23
–, –, –, γ genes 23
–, –, –, low density lipoprotein (LDL) receptor
    24
–, –, –, structure 23
–, –, –, synthesis 28

–, –, C8′ 21
–, –, C8α 22
–, –, –, functional domain on α 22
–, –, –, α-helical transmembrane segments 24
–, –, –, membrane surface-seeking segments 24
–, –, C8β 21
–, –, –, amino acid sequence of human β 24
–, –, –, functional domains on β 21
–, –, –, topology 21
–, –, C8γ 23
–, –, –, functional domains on γ 23
–, –, –, "lipocalins" 26
–, –, –, sequence of human γ 26
–, –, C9 19, 34
–, –, –, amphipathic helix 58
–, –, –, domain 52
–, –, –, gene 50
–, –, –, polymerization 112
–, –, –, polymers 60
–, –, –, protein 50
–, –, –, surface features 53
conjugates 1
CTL activation 74
cytodot 69
cytotoxicity 33
–, α1-antichymotrypsin 33
–, α1-antitrypsin 33
–, correlations 88
–, –, serine protease inhibitor 89
–, DFP-inactivation 33
–, PMSF-inactivation 33

DAF 110
delivery, P1-mediated 5
DNA degradation 4

esterase, acetylcholine 110
exon-intron organization 72
expression 43
–, mRNA 11

function, granzymes 44
–, – A 44
–, structure 44

genes, CTL-specific 68
–, function related 68
granules 34
–, cytolytic 2, 12
–, cytoplasmic 72
–, secretory 96, 97
granzymes 35

"Hanukah factor" (HF) 82
– –, cleavage specificities 82
– –, expression 84
– –, –, anomalous 86
– –, –, CD4⁻CD8⁺T-cells 87
– –, human 83
– –, –, CTLs 83
– –, serine protease cascade 83, 89–90
homologous restriction factor (HRF)
    114
– species restriction 110
homology 39
–, catalytic site 40
–, cathepsin G 39
–, granzyme B 39
–, propeptide 40
–, rat mast cell protease II 39
–, signal peptide 40
hybridization, in situ 86, 69

inhibitors 33
–, aprotinin 37
–, benzamidine 37
–, DFP 37
–, leupeptin 37
–, PMSF 37
–, TLCK 37
–, TPCK 37
"innocent bystander lysis" 116

killer cell reorientation 2

lipoprotein 116
lymphocytes, activated cytotoxic T (CTLs)
    81
lysis, CTL-mediated 76
–, innocent bystander 116

mast cells 44
membrane attack complexes 49
molecular biology, secretory granule proteogly-
    cans 97

NK cells 102, 103
Northern blot 39

paroxysmal nocturnal hemoglobinuria
    (PNH) III
perforin 11, 28, 55
perforin 1, 3
– complex, poly 11
perforin/cytolysin 34
peritoneal exudate cells 7
phosphatidylinositol-specific phospholipase C
    (PIPLC) (PI) 110
PNH-E 112
polyadenylyation 39
–, signal peptide 39
protease cascade 70
proteases, serine 33, 70
S-protein 61
protein, adhesion 1
–, granular 76
proteoglycans 93
–, biochemistry 94

regions, DNase-sensitive 76
rejections, allograft 86

secretion, vectorial granule 1
secretory machinery 2
serine protease 82
– –, signal sequence 70
– – genes, cytotoxic-T-lymphocytes-specific
    67 ff
serotonin 116
similarities, structural, between α, β, γ and
    C9 27
–, –, –, perforin 28
sorting 43
Southern blot 39
specificity, substrate 43, 72
S-protein 61, 113, 116
structure, tertiary 41
subfamily, granzyme 41
–, –, chondroitin sulfate 41
–, –, disulfide bridges 41
–, –, glycosylation 41
–, serine protease 73
substrates, granzyme D 37
–, Pro-Phe-Arg-7-amino-4-methyl-coumarin 37
–, Pro-Phe-Arg-nitroanilide 37
–, Succ-Ala-Phe-Lys 37
sulfate, chondroitin 6
synthesis, thromboxane 116

T cells, cytotoxic 1
thromboxane synthesis 116
transmembrane pores 1

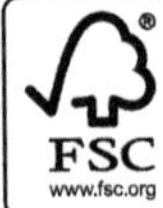

If you have any concerns about our products,
you can contact us on
ProductSafety@springernature.com

In case Publisher is established outside the EU,
the EU authorized representative is:
Springer Nature Customer Service Center GmbH
Europaplatz 3, 69115 Heidelberg, Germany

Printed by Libri Plureos GmbH
in Hamburg, Germany